Live Your Best Life

DK

Live Your Best Life

219 Science-Based Reasons to Rethink Your Daily Routine

DR. STUART FARRIMOND

Project Editor Francesco Piscitelli
Project Designer Simon Murrell
Senior Editor Rona Skene
US Editor Jennette ElNaggar
Project Art Editor Louise Brigenshaw
Illustrators Mik Gates, Mark Clifton
Designer Natalie Clay
Editorial Assistant Kiron Gill
Senior Jackets Creative Nicola Powling
Pre-production Producer David Almond
Senior Producer Luca Bazzoli
Creative Technical Support Tom Morse
Managing Editor Dawn Henderson
Managing Art Editor Marianne Markham
Art Director Maxine Pedliham
Publishing Director Mary-Clare Jerram

First American Edition, 2020
Published in the United States by DK Publishing
1450 Broadway, Suite 801, New York, NY 10018

DISCLAIMER see page 256

A catalog record for this book is available
from the Library of Congress.
ISBN 978-1-4654-9329-3

Printed and bound in China

For the curious

www.dk.com

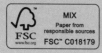

CONTENTS

EVENING 146

Foreword

"Science." If the word brings to mind dreary lessons, mumbo-jumbo jargon, and bookish bores who are no fun at a party, then this book is for you. All too often we think that science means distilling our world into dry numbers and equations. In reality, science gives richness, meaning, and depth to our daily lives. In seven years in medicine, not only did I learn the intricacies of the human body and the diseases that afflict it, but I was molded into the role of a doctor and taught to skillfully hide behind a cloak of jargon and science-speak. Only after stepping back from the profession did I discover how truly alienated we academic types can make others feel. Much of this highbrow babble does nothing but separate us from others. This book seeks to set the record straight and show that you do not need letters after your name to understand life's little mysteries.

Every day brings with it countless questions. Not just the philosophical ones but also momentary wonderings—should I drink a coffee first thing in the morning or wait awhile? Why are there so many bad drivers on the road? Why do I feel so sluggish after lunch? Newspaper columns and clickbait websites are filled with pithy answers to such questions. Many of these explanations leave us wanting. They may sound reasonable, but sometimes they're misleading or just plain wrong.

Dozens of specialists and experts from around the world helped me craft this book, which represents the most up-to-date science and research that answers these questions. Rather than serve you up feel-good self-help fluff with every answer, I hope to explain the science in a way that everybody will understand and so be empowered to make better decisions.

I take you through a typical day—morning, afternoon, evening, and night—answering those "I wonder why?" questions when they are most likely to crop up. Of course, not everything fits neatly into a time slot, and you may do things at different times; for example, some prefer to exercise at the crack of dawn, others in the evening. I hope this helps you navigate through your day. I have also tried to make the book relevant, regardless of your age, gender, race, creed, and culture.

Above all, this book is a celebration of life. It is the most precious thing we have. Life deserves to be filled with laughter, love, kindness, and passion. Yet it is desperately fragile. I think that we only really appreciate just how wonderful life is when we go face-to-face with the reality that ours will one day come to an end. It is only when we realize that our existence is but a grain of sand in the infinity of time that we learn to truly relish every day we have on planet Earth. The COVID-19 pandemic has brought this uncomfortable truth into sharp focus to all of us. During the writing of this book, I have endured surgery, radiotherapy, and chemotherapy for what has now become an aggressive brain cancer. It is with the steadfast love and support of family and friends that I have learned to love life. Writing this book has helped me live life to its fullest. I hope that in reading it, it helps you live yours to the fullest, too.

Stuart Farrimond

MORNING

Nature really has no sense of manners. Starting before sunrise, birds tweet and warble at a volume loud enough to unsettle even the heaviest sleeper. Just like our feathered neighbors, we have a body clock that wakes us in the morning. At its command, our internal systems flutter into life and our brain steadily becomes primed to focus on the day's business. You may not have the sparkle of a sparrow, but the same energizing hormones flood through your blood, enabling you to fly headlong into the new day.

Why Is Waking Up So Hard?

Many body systems, from the digestive tract to the thinking regions of your brain, rest as you sleep. Getting the motors running again can be like starting a car on a frosty morning.

When you sleep, your body cycles repeatedly through a natural rhythm of sleep stages. If you are lucky enough to wake during a good dream (during an REM stage), expect to wake energized. However, if you wake from deep, dreamless sleep (during a non-REM stage), you will probably feel groggy, starting the day with the mental vigor of a slug.

When you wake suddenly from deep sleep, rather than rising naturally

70% OF PEOPLE EXPERIENCE **SLEEP INERTIA** FOR THE **FIRST HOUR OR TWO** OF THEIR DAY

(see page 15), the frontal thinking parts of your brain aren't ready to spark into life; instead, they are straining to shift into normal thinking activities. This brain lag is called sleep inertia and has several effects: your reaction times are terrible, thinking and reasoning are muddy, and memory is at its worst. You will also suffer worse sleep inertia if you're sleep deprived—and sprightly morning larks aren't immune to its effects, either.

Sleep inertia is common, but thankfully it's temporary and lasts for only the first hour or two of the day. There are techniques (see left) that you can try to ease its effects.

FEELING GROGGY THIS MORNING?

1

GET OUT INTO DAYLIGHT to kick-start your body clock and boost levels of "wake-up" hormones (see pages 22–23).

2

TRY STRETCHING, YOGA, AND GENTLE EXERCISE, such as a brisk walk or bike ride—these all increase your heart rate, improve blood flow to the parts of your brain that are still "asleep," and boost your mood.

3

DON'T MAKE BIG DECISIONS because you won't make the best choices, even if you think you're clear-headed.

REACTION
TIMES ARE
360%
SLOWER

ABILITY
TO PROCESS
INFORMATION IS
70%
SLOWER

ABILITY
TO MAKE GOOD
DECISIONS IS
51%
WORSE

EFFECTS OF SLEEP
INERTIA

SLOW START

People who are abruptly awoken and
experience sleep inertia have lowered
reaction times and decision-making abilities.
In several studies, most cognitive functions
were impaired immediately after waking.

Why Do I Feel Low on Winter Mornings?

If a miserable mood seems to go hand in glove with short, chilly winter days, then you aren't alone; many people are more sleepy and have less energy during wintertime.

Some scientists think that during darker, winter days, a lack of sunlight hitting the eyes tricks your body clock into generating an excess of its natural sleep hormone melatonin, vaporizing your regular happy sparkle. However, other studies have cast doubt on this theory, by showing that people living in polar regions who face dark days for half the year don't tend to suffer from persistent low mood. This may be because they make a conscious effort to socialize and maintain their regular activities. If harsh weather prevents you from exercising or seeing loved ones and keeps you cooped up indoors like a hibernating bear, then your mental well-being will almost certainly take a hit.

If you suffer winter blues, light therapy—a daily dose of artificial light—has been shown to be effective. And perhaps if we take a lead from the Scandinavians, who see cold seasons as a chance to see more of friends and family, we may feel less gloomy at the onset of winter.

80% OF SAD SYMPTOMS IMPROVE AFTER EARLY MORNING LIGHT THERAPY

38% OF SAD SYMPTOMS IMPROVE AFTER LATE MORNING LIGHT THERAPY

30% OF SAD SYMPTOMS IMPROVE AFTER EVENING LIGHT THERAPY

LET THERE BE LIGHT
Research shows that, for most people diagnosed with seasonal affective disorder (SAD), light therapy is most beneficial if taken for 30 minutes immediately after waking.

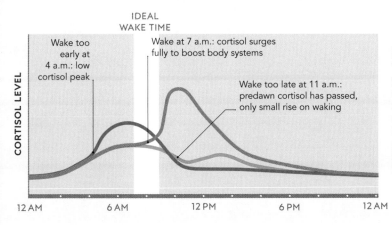

I Slept In, So Why Do I Still Feel Sleepy?

When you wake after a longer-than-usual night's sleep,
you expect to feel refreshed, so it's baffling when instead
you feel even worse than on a normal morning.

Your body has a fixed sleep-wake rhythm (see pages 22–23), and it starts to rev up your biological engines way in advance of the ordeal of waking. Long before your natural waking time, the powerful energizing hormone cortisol is released into your blood in increasing amounts. Cortisol boosts energy and motivation and increases the level of blood sugar in order to fuel the brain and muscles and get you moving. The moment you wake up, cortisol surges even further, helping to hurl you into the land of the living. If you sleep through your early morning cortisol buzz, the normally invigorating hormone ebbs away uselessly, and you don't have its energizing benefits when you do wake. This is why sleeping in on the weekend can actually leave you feeling worse than an early start on a workday.

It is possible to catch up on some lost sleep on the weekend, but you can expect to reclaim only half of the deficit (see page 231). It's best to go to bed and wake up at the same time every day so that your body clock can naturally take you through the morning.

Should I Hit the Snooze Button?

The most effective alarms are noisy and harsh. They are foolproof because they trigger a primal bodily fear response. In short, they give you a touch of morning terror.

That loud morning buzzer triggers instinctive survival responses in an area deep in the brain called the amygdala. Your heart rate soars as cortisol (see page 15) and the fight-or-flight hormone adrenaline stream through the body—just in case you need to run for your life. Clearly, there is no wild beast about to pounce, and when your conscious mind realizes this, the adrenaline surge fades and you may doze off again. But hit the snooze button, and you are about to add insult to injury. An extra 10–15 minutes simply is not long enough for you to be able to sink back into a refreshing sleep. When the alarm shocks you awake, you suffer the same biological torment all over again. Repeated surges of fear-fueled adrenaline may well force you out of bed but over time can put your mood on a downer and affect your physical health; years of stressful wakenings actually contribute to the clogging of blood vessels, which can in turn increase the risk of heart problems.

It's best to set the alarm for your desired waking time, then get up right away. If you really want that extra snooze, allow yourself at least 45 minutes to reap some benefit. Or see the box on the left for tips to help reduce your reliance on the dreaded alarm.

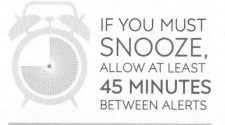

IF YOU MUST **SNOOZE,** ALLOW AT LEAST **45 MINUTES** BETWEEN ALERTS

WANT TO **BEAT THE ALARM?**

1
LEAVE THE CURTAINS OPEN OVERNIGHT to allow daylight into your bedroom as early as possible; sensors in the back of the eye detect the dawn through your eyelids, priming the body clock for morning.

2
SET THE CENTRAL HEATING to come on at least half an hour before you wake, to mimic the temperature change as the sun rises.

3
RIG A TIME SWITCH TO YOUR BEDSIDE LAMP and fit a "daylight" bulb; set it for half an hour before the alarm to jump-start the cortisol surge.

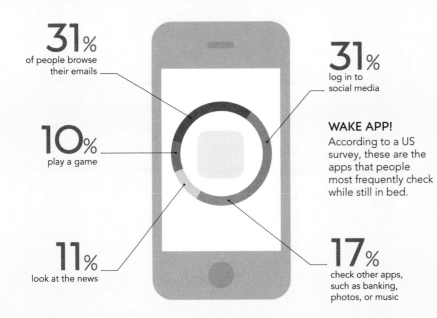

31% of people browse their emails

31% log in to social media

10% play a game

WAKE APP!
According to a US survey, these are the apps that people most frequently check while still in bed.

11% look at the news

17% check other apps, such as banking, photos, or music

Is It Okay to Check My Phone As Soon As I Wake?

It's no wonder we can't resist—with news, emails, games, and social media, our smartphones are a mental Aladdin's cave. But is swiping and tapping really the best start to the day?

You're vulnerable when you first wake up—the logical, thinking parts of your brain take a while to become fully awake, and you're less able to make good decisions, handle new information, and solve problems. Open apps such as emails and to-do lists in the first hour, and you risk getting out of bed on the wrong side, as research shows that these can trigger anxiety.

Your focus then quickly becomes blinkered, further muddying your shaky morning judgment and potentially pushing up your already-surging cortisol to unhealthy peaks.

If you're a first-thing phone-checker, consider moving troubling apps away from your home screen. Fill these prime spots instead with apps that offer relaxing or uplifting content.

Why Don't I Remember My Dreams?

Your dreams have more excitement, emotion, and terror than any Hollywood blockbuster, but unfortunately, your brain switches off its memory stores at night.

Everyone dreams—even the 5 percent who say they never do. Almost all of your dreams happen when in a stage of sleep called REM (also known as rapid eye movement). During this stage, much of your brain is very active, almost exactly as if you were awake. Come sunrise, though, usually most memories of your dreams will have mysteriously vanished.

25%
—THE **PROPORTION** OF A TOTAL NIGHT'S **DREAMS** THAT WE ARE **ABLE TO RECALL**

When you dream, your memory storage capabilities, centered around a brain region called the hippocampus, are dialed right back—so most of your bizarre nighttime experiences are as fleeting as a shooting star. It seems to be that the hippocampus opts not to store most dreams because it deems them irrelevant compared to the real events that are worth remembering in your waking life. However, people (including young children) who might attach significance to their dreams are more likely to remember them.

If you wake up during REM sleep, then you will probably be able to describe what was happening in your dream at that very moment. Your memory circuitry will still be sluggish at that time, so to help embed dreams in your longer-term memory, record them on a notepad or phone right away before they fade. Studies show that the act of recording your dream helps you recall visual details.

You can also increase your chances of recalling dreams by timing your alarm to go off in the REM stage and make it more likely that you'll wake up mid-dream.

If you can't remember your dreams, there's no cause for worry—it just shows that your brain is giving your memory a much-needed rest.

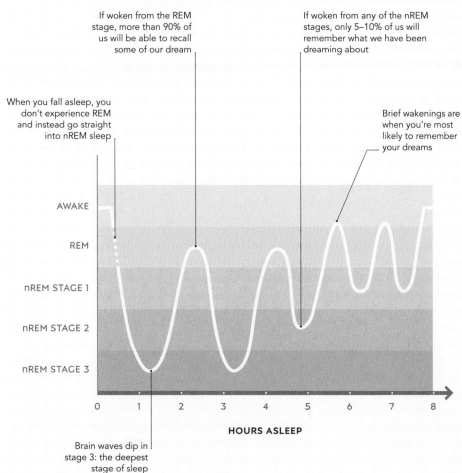

If woken from the REM stage, more than 90% of us will be able to recall some of our dream

If woken from any of the nREM stages, only 5–10% of us will remember what we have been dreaming about

When you fall asleep, you don't experience REM and instead go straight into nREM sleep

Brief wakenings are when you're most likely to remember your dreams

AWAKE

REM

nREM STAGE 1

nREM STAGE 2

nREM STAGE 3

STAGES OF SLEEP

0   1   2   3   4   5   6   7   8

HOURS ASLEEP

Brain waves dip in stage 3: the deepest stage of sleep

SURFING THE BRAIN WAVES

When you sleep, brain waves dip in and out of four different stages. Most of your sleep (75–80 percent) is spent in the calm, restorative non-REM stages, while the rest you spend in REM, where most of your dreams occur. You're much more likely to remember your dreams if you wake from REM sleep.

When Should I Drink My First Coffee?

If you reach for a cup of coffee first thing in the morning, then count yourself as one of the millions who use caffeine to kick-start their day. But does it help or hinder you?

Caffeine is a powerful stimulant. It speeds up thinking, boosts motivation, and lifts mood, but it does so by temporarily blocking one of the body's naturally calming brain hormones—adenosine. Within 10 minutes of slurping your early-morning beverage, caffeine is coursing through your blood and sets to work on your brain by blocking adenosine. But the problem is that, at this time, the energizing hormone cortisol is at its peak, while adenosine is at its lowest. A strong coffee or tea on top of all that cortisol doesn't make you more alert—it simply throws a few matches onto an already raging bonfire, increasing your chances of anxiety and jitteriness. Your espresso is worse than pointless.

You're much better off waiting a few hours until cortisol has waned and adenosine has started to rise, and then you can reap the full benefit of caffeine's boost.

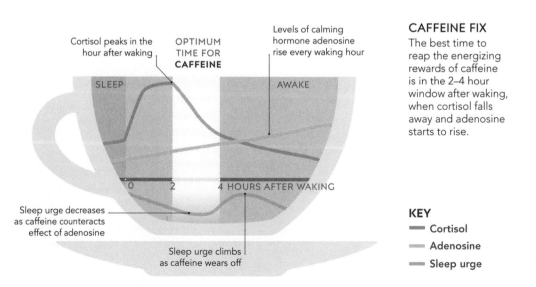

Cortisol peaks in the hour after waking

OPTIMUM TIME FOR CAFFEINE

Levels of calming hormone adenosine rise every waking hour

SLEEP

AWAKE

0   2   4 HOURS AFTER WAKING

Sleep urge decreases as caffeine counteracts effect of adenosine

Sleep urge climbs as caffeine wears off

CAFFEINE FIX
The best time to reap the energizing rewards of caffeine is in the 2–4 hour window after waking, when cortisol falls away and adenosine starts to rise.

KEY
— Cortisol
— Adenosine
— Sleep urge

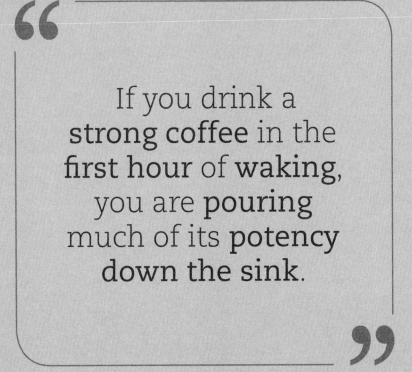

" If you drink a **strong coffee** in the **first hour** of **waking**, you are **pouring** much of its **potency** down the sink. "

Can I Make Myself More of a Morning Person?

Studies show that the most successful people are early risers. CEOs and highfliers swear by waking up before 5 a.m., but for many, getting up at that hour is simply torture.

Some of us bounce out of bed in the morning; others recoil at the blinding morning sun. The idea that there are "morning" or "evening" people is much more than an urban myth. Everyone has a body clock timetable (chronotype) that controls when they naturally wake, eat, work, play, and sleep, but the exact timings are different for each of us. A small proportion of us are primed to fire on all cylinders as soon as the sun rises ("morning larks"). Nearly a quarter of us are energized around sundown ("night owls"). The rest fly somewhere down the middle. Unfortunately, for owls, studies show that larks generally do better than them at school, live longer, and earn on average 5 percent more.

However, forcing yourself to be an early riser isn't a good idea—night owls' shorter life expectancy may be due to the biological strain of trying to live by a strict 9–5 work culture. Thankfully, the option of flexible work times is becoming more widely available to workers, and the owl-lark income divide is narrowing.

Although you can't change your chronotype, you can work with it to get more out of your day. If you are a night owl, try to shift your routine to fit your natural energy levels. If you have no option but to get up early, try daytime napping—even 20 minutes during the post-lunch slump can be restorative. Consider also that some lifestyles and careers are actually better suited to night owls; for example, those working in hospitality or entertainment, or evening shift workers, will all be more successful if they are natural late risers.

21% OF ADULTS
ARE **NIGHT OWLS** AND ABOUT **14%** ARE **LARKS**

WHAT IS THE BODY CLOCK?

Your body clock is a tiny bundle of nerves called the suprachiasmatic nucleus (SCN) about the size of a pinhead, buried in the underside of your brain. Signals from specialized daylight-sensing cells in the eyes alert the SCN to release hormones that send messages to all body systems.

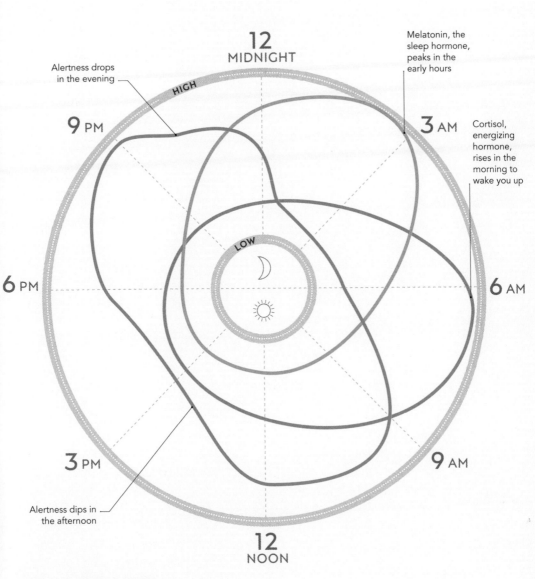

12
MIDNIGHT

Alertness drops
in the evening

HIGH

9 PM

Melatonin, the
sleep hormone,
peaks in the
early hours

3 AM

Cortisol,
energizing
hormone,
rises in the
morning to
wake you up

6 PM

LOW

6 AM

3 PM

9 AM

Alertness dips in
the afternoon

12
NOON

HORMONES IN CHARGE

The body clock is the conductor of your internal
systems. The release of different amounts of
hormones melatonin and cortisol at various times
affects your mental and physical alertness
throughout the day. This clock shows the hormone
level of somebody who's neither a lark nor an owl.

KEY
— Cortisol
— Melatonin
— Alertness

Why Are Teenagers So Lazy in the Mornings?

You can blame them for a messy bedroom, but you can't scold teens for their reluctance to get out of bed in the morning—their body clocks are changing.

During the tumultuous teen years, hormones are surging and the body is changing dramatically. Meanwhile, large swathes of the brain are rewiring (see pages 118–119).

One of the side effects of this biological turmoil is that a teenager's body clock moves forward. As a result, they become more inclined to go to sleep later and also wake up later. They aren't just being lazy—their body really is in a different time zone! For a typical 16-year-old, 10 p.m. feels like your 8 p.m., and a 7 a.m. alarm carries the pain of an adult's 5 a.m. disturbance.

No one knows exactly why the adolescent's body clock makes this two-hour shift, but it's an inescapable result of the child brain maturing into an adult one. Interestingly, similar changes happen after puberty in other animals, including monkeys and mice.

When a teenager lives in a world of 8:30 a.m. starts, they will become progressively more sleep deprived—going to sleep late yet still being forced to get up at "adult time." When the weekend comes, it's normal for teenagers to have marathon sleep-ins to try to compensate.

A teenager's brain tends to be foggier during the morning, so some schools have experimented with later start times and moving the most mentally taxing subjects to later in the day. This has generally proved successful, with attendance rates, sickness, and academic performance all improving.

So go easy on teens—for a number of years, they will be going through a perpetual jet lag of sorts. The body clock is at its latest when you get to 20, and thereafter it slides back with each passing year.

STUDIES SHOW THAT **STARTING** THE **SCHOOL DAY** AN **HOUR LATER** IMPROVES TEENS'
ACHIEVEMENT BY 10%

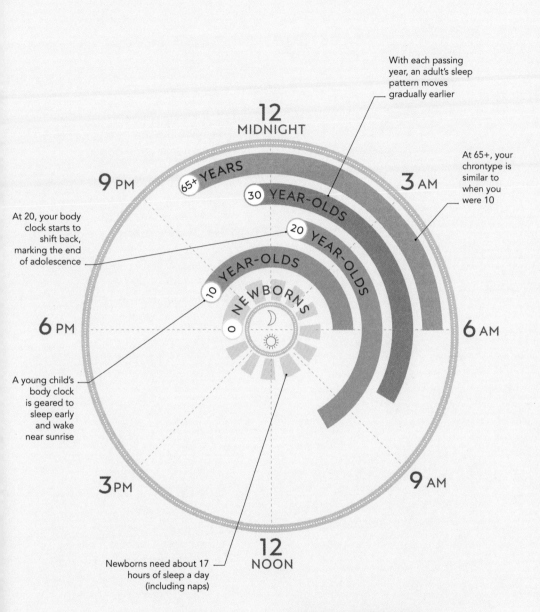

With each passing year, an adult's sleep pattern moves gradually earlier

At 65+, your chrontype is similar to when you were 10

12 MIDNIGHT

9 PM

3 AM

65+ YEARS

30 YEAR-OLDS

20 YEAR-OLDS

At 20, your body clock starts to shift back, marking the end of adolescence

YEAR-OLDS

NEWBORNS

6 PM

0

6 AM

A young child's body clock is geared to sleep early and wake near sunrise

3 PM

9 AM

12 NOON

Newborns need about 17 hours of sleep a day (including naps)

SHIFTING SLEEP TIMES

As you age, your body clock shifts back and forth. For most of your life, you tend to go to sleep between 9–11 p.m. and wake at sunrise. However, throughout the teen years, the body clock temporarily changes to run much later.

When Is the Best Time to Shower or Bathe?

Most of us wash every day, and we have our preferred methods, but how and when you do should really depend on whether you're revving up or winding down.

For a morning wake-up call, a cold shower is usually best—a splash of chilly water over the body makes levels of cortisol and adrenaline surge briefly, giving as much punch as a caffeine hit. If stepping into an icy-cold shower first thing is just unbearable, try ending a warm shower with a 30-second blast of cold water. This will deliver an invigorating boost and—according to one large study—it will even make it less likely that you'll take time off sick from work.

STAY **CLEAN AND FRESH**

1
TAKE A COLD SHOWER in the morning to give both body and mind a wake-up boost.

2
TAKE A HOT SHOWER OR BATH in the evening to calm your mind so that you prepare for sleep.

3
BATHE OR SHOWER no more than once a day so that you don't wash away your skin and hair's natural oils.

If a good night's sleep is your goal, then a warm shower or bath about 90 minutes before bed is highly effective in helping the body and brain wind down—this lowers blood pressure; stimulates the release of the positive, happiness hormone serotonin; lowers anxiety levels; and can make cortisol levels plunge by a third. A cold shower has the opposite effect so is best avoided late in the evenings.

Of course, you might think that you can cash in on all the benefits with a morning shower and an evening bath. Rinse that thought—dermatologists say that twice-a-day bathing is probably too much. Your skin and hair are coated in a barely visible sheen of an oily substance called sebum. This is your body's natural waterproof gloss, and it's constantly replenished via microscopic pores in your skin. Washing twice a day scrubs away the skin's sebum, and without it your skin will dry out and become sore, chapped, or infected. Bath lovers, beware—long, hot soaks in a tub of bubbles feels luxurious, but it's best to shower or bathe for only about 5–10 minutes in lukewarm water every two or three days to give time for sebum to replenish itself.

In our overly washed and manicured world, skin and hair can become so depleted of their natural oils that we think we need moisturizing creams and lotions to restore their luster. Much of what you might slather over yourself is, however, nothing more than nice-smelling grease. Moisturizers don't actually "moisturize"—they simply replace the oily protective coat that

STRESS HORMONE
CORTISOL PLUNGES BY A THIRD WHEN YOU'RE IMMERSED IN **HOT WATER**

you wash down the plughole with your soap or shampoo. Added "skin nourishing" ingredients emblazoned on the packaging are mostly marketing froth that have little added effect. Similarly, hair conditioners are merely a replacement for the natural oils that the body freely makes. If you shower or bathe every two or three days, you likely won't need skin moisturizers or hair conditioners.

SINGING IN THE SHOWER IS GOOD FOR YOU!

As the bathroom mirror steams up, an audience of silent yellow rubber ducks stare in awe at your rendition of "Fly Me to the Moon." Frank Sinatra never sounded this good—at least to your own ears!

Emotions and music are knotted in your brain tighter than the mess of cables behind your television. You really do "feel" music because the emotional areas of your brain (called the limbic system) become active when you sing cheery songs.

Also, you genuinely sound better in your bathroom: the tiled surfaces echo vocal pitches back and forth, reverberating each crooning note to last slightly longer, smoothing out a wobbly voice, and masking any off notes. You're also louder, which no doubt helps boost your mood even further. Some artists have even made commercial recordings in their bathroom because the acoustics are so good.

Your soapy serenade will also be deeper and throatier in the morning. While you haven't been speaking overnight, your vocal cords relax themselves, much like a guitarist might release the tension from their guitar's string.

It's such a pity the duckies are the only ones to realize just how great a singer you truly are....

Why Do I Poop at the Same Time Every Morning?

Just like the rest of your body, the digestive system obeys the ticktock of your internal clock. As you become active during the first few hours after waking, so does your gut.

Most of us have our main bowel movement in the morning because the digestive system "sleeps" at night and reawakens according to our body clock (see pages 22–23). Strong, muscular contractions (called the migrating motor complex) ripple through the intestines to push out waste, making space for the coming day's food intake. Similar contractions may happen throughout the day.

Your gut's unique routine is shaped by your body clock, lifestyle, and diet. "Regular" for you can be anything between three times a day and three times a week. Having a lifestyle that

EATING **30G** OF **FIBER** PER DAY KEEPS YOUR GUT **REGULAR** AND **HEALTHY**

is off-kilter with your body clock (such as working night shifts) may mean that this major morning emptying doesn't happen, is less regular, or just happens at a different time of day.

Regular bowel movements go hand in hand with a healthy gut, and this is important for overall health. Hormones from the gut affect your emotions, your immune system, your energy levels, and blood sugar control.

Fiber, carbohydrates, fats, protein, and fluids all play their part in keeping digesting food moving easily, and any diet that focuses on, or cuts out, one of these groups is a good recipe for clogged piping. See the panel to the left for some tips to show your gut some love and stay regular.

HELP YOUR **GUT**

1

EAT FOODS WITH FIBER to add bulk that the intestines can push against, and drink plenty of water to lubricate your gut.

2

GOING FOR A WALK or any light exercise will stimulate blood flow to the intestines and help the gut run smoothly.

EXHALED BREATH

Smells like feces

Smells like dead animals

Smells like sweaty feet

NOXIOUS MIX
As microbes digest food particles, they produce various foul-smelling chemicals.

MICROBES IN THE MOUTH

Why Do I Have Bad Breath When I Wake Up?

Come daybreak, even lovingly flossed pearly whites may end up feeling "furry" and your breath smelling funky. The culprits are the mob of microbes that live in your mouth.

During the day, glands in the cheeks and mouth produce an astonishing one quart of saliva, which contains an armada of microbe-killing molecules alongside tooth-protecting chemicals that clump nasty microbes into harmless flotsam. When you're asleep, this flow reduces to a tiny trickle and your mouth runs dry, allowing microbes to proliferate and latch onto your teeth—creating a fuzzy film called plaque. As they feast on traces of food and sugar left from the day, they emit foul-smelling gases that cause malodorous morning breath. Sleeping with an open mouth makes the problem even worse, so your breath will smell if your nose is blocked by a cold or hay fever.

Brushing your teeth helps (minty toothpastes mask the smell) and having breakfast early stimulates saliva production. Ironically, testosterone peaks in the morning, making you amorous just when getting up close is least appealing: nature truly does have a mischievous sense of humor!

What's the Best Toothpaste for Healthy Teeth?

Everyone knows that brushing twice a day is the cornerstone of good dental health, so why exactly do you need toothpaste—and what's the best one to use?

Most of us firmly believe that regular brushing with toothpaste is essential to prevent plaque buildup on our teeth and to keep tooth decay at bay. Dental experts have told us this for over a century, so there's no reason to doubt it, right? Not so.

The truth is that neither toothpaste in itself nor the act of brushing are what primarily prevents tooth decay—it's the magic ingredient, fluoride, that achieves this by soaking through the gums and strengthening tooth enamel.

The main driver for tooth decay is not plaque but what you eat. Long before toothpaste, and before humans started milling flour to make bread, cakes, and noodles, tooth decay was as rare as hen's teeth. Today, a typical diet is high in refined carbohydrates and sugars, which supercharge microbes in your mouth to spew out acids that will erode enamel.

Fluoride definitely prevents decay, but so-called "whitening" toothpastes won't make your teeth gleam—they may get rid of some yellowish staining, but just don't expect a movie star sparkle. Some contain questionably effective abrasive ingredients that break down or soak up stains; others employ chemicals that provide only

If your toothpaste has no fluoride in it, you're at risk of cavities

0 PPM

1,000–1,250 PPM

1,450–1,500 PPM

Low fluoride levels offer some protection

Ideal level of fluoride to provide good protection

FLUORIDE FLAWS

Fluoride is the most important ingredient in toothpastes because it prevents tooth decay. The fluoride content in a toothpaste is measured in PPM (parts per million).

a temporary whitening effect. No matter how much you scrub, you'll never restore your teeth to the color of a baby's teeth, though; enamel slowly and inevitably thins as we get older, revealing more of the yellowish layer called dentin underneath.

TOOTHPASTES WITH ADDED FLUORIDE PREVENT 25% OF CAVITIES THAT WOULD OTHERWISE FORM

Some toothpastes aimed at those with sensitive teeth do actually work—they temporarily clog up microscopic holes within dentin that cause pain when eating ice cream or drinking cold drinks.

TOOTHPASTE TIPS

1
USE FLUORIDE TOOTHPASTE and let the fluoride absorb fully in the mouth by spitting, not rinsing, the toothpaste after brushing.

2
BRUSH REGULARLY in a gentle motion, to clean gums without damaging them.

3
DON'T USE MOUTHWASH within 30 minutes of brushing as it will wash away toothpaste, reducing fluoride.

THE GRIMY TOOTHPASTE CON

The idea that toothpaste can strip away plaque didn't come from a scientist but from an American businessman, Claude Hopkins, who worked for the US toothpaste company Pepsodent in the early 1900s. Until then, toothpaste was sold as a cosmetic product for keeping teeth looking whiter for longer, although it wasn't even very good at doing that.

Without any scientific evidence, the marketing maestro crafted an advertising campaign around the catchy but inaccurate idea that Pepsodent could remove a "film" on the teeth that caused dullness and gum disease. The toothpaste was claimed to contain a decay-fighting ingredient called "irium"—an impressively scientific-sounding name that is now known to be merely Hopkins's alternative name for the frothing agent sodium lauryl sulphate. Even though experts lambasted the campaign as quackery, the public was won over, and the product became a runaway success worldwide.

The lofty claims had no substance—Pepsodent was just as ineffective at preventing tooth decay as any of its rivals. In fact, it wasn't until fluoride was added to toothpaste, decades later, that it did anything other than make a nice froth and leave a minty taste.

Is an Electric Toothbrush the Best Way to Brush?

Electric toothbrushes are a common fixture in our bathrooms—but are they really a better bet than old-fashioned arm power or just a gadget-lover's fad?

Advertisements often proclaim that "most dental hygienists recommend an electric toothbrush." However, much of this research has been done by those with skin in the game—namely, the toothbrush manufacturers themselves—so should not be swallowed whole. An unbiased look at the science proves that some electric toothbrushes do indeed give a more thorough clean when used correctly, although the extra plaque-scrubbing

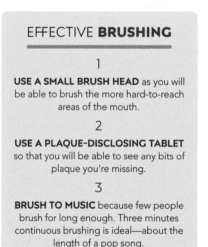

21% LESS
PLAQUE REMAINED AFTER BRUSHING WITH AN **ELECTRIC TOOTHBRUSH** COMPARED TO USING A **REGULAR TOOTHBRUSH**

power is not as vast as the companies that sell these products would have you believe.

Devices with heads that spin one way and then the other ("rotation-oscillation") are the best of the bunch. Claims made for other "ultrasonic" heads that vibrate at extremely high speeds are on much shakier ground and are likely to be more spin than substance. If you do use an electric toothbrush, remember that you don't have to scrub. The spinning head is putting in the elbow grease and brushing for you, so the bristles just need to be moved over and in between all the tooth surfaces. Pressing down too hard actually risks scraping off some of the tooth's enamel.

EFFECTIVE **BRUSHING**

1

USE A SMALL BRUSH HEAD as you will be able to brush the more hard-to-reach areas of the mouth.

2

USE A PLAQUE-DISCLOSING TABLET so that you will be able to see any bits of plaque you're missing.

3

BRUSH TO MUSIC because few people brush for long enough. Three minutes continuous brushing is ideal—about the length of a pop song.

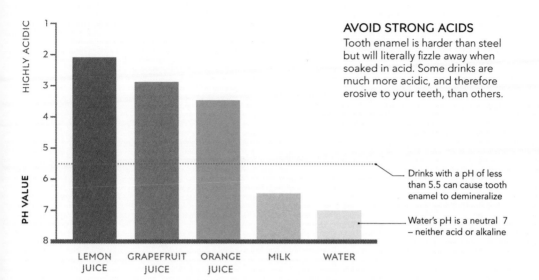

AVOID STRONG ACIDS
Tooth enamel is harder than steel but will literally fizzle away when soaked in acid. Some drinks are much more acidic, and therefore erosive to your teeth, than others.

HIGHLY ACIDIC

PH VALUE

1 — 2 — 3 — 4 — 5 — 6 — 7 — 8

Drinks with a pH of less than 5.5 can cause tooth enamel to demineralize

Water's pH is a neutral 7 – neither acid or alkaline

LEMON JUICE · GRAPEFRUIT JUICE · ORANGE JUICE · MILK · WATER

Should I Brush My Teeth Before or After Breakfast?

Brushing after sweeps away food remnants from breakfast, whereas brushing before gets rid of morning breath, but is one option better than the other?

Brushing your teeth after eating is fine, but there are drawbacks, depending on what you had for breakfast. Acids in certain food and drinks temporarily soften enamel, the tooth's shiny outer coating. Substances in our saliva neutralize these acids, although this can take up to an hour.

If you brush during this vulnerable window, you risk scrubbing off enamel. Over time, this erosion puts you at risk of developing cavities (crevices where bacteria can breed). Brushing before eating creates its own, albeit less serious, issue: toothpaste's foaming agent—sodium lauryl sulphate (SLS)—wreaks havoc on your taste buds, blocking the tongue's ability to taste sweetness and leaving an unpleasant, bitter taste that is especially pronounced when you drink citrus juice.

Is Breakfast the Most Important Meal of the Day?

You might think of this mantra as one handed down through the generations, but in reality, it's a modern invention that's based more on sales than in science.

Breakfast wasn't always the institution it is today. The ancient Romans, for instance, would eat just one substantial meal in the middle of the day, snacking lightly at dawn and dusk.

In more recent history, US breakfast cereal manufacturers initially promoted their wares as a healthy alternative for a population who ate badly. Their advertising campaigns reinforced the importance of breakfast—and catchy slogans such as "eat breakfast like a king" by Adelle Davis, a US celebrity nutritionist whose advice is now considered spurious, sealed the deal. The veneration of breakfast is still felt in the zeitgeist today—especially in Western countries.

Modern studies show that eating breakfast doesn't "kick-start" your body's metabolism (the rate at which you burn calories). There is a small rise in metabolic rate after any meal due to

AFTER 8 HOURS WITHOUT FOOD, MOST OF THE **ENERGY STORED** IN THE **LIVER** HAS BEEN **USED UP**

the energy needed to digest food—but it is no more marked at breakfast than at any other meal.

Your body clock (see pages 22–23) will determine whether you need or want breakfast. Given that the ebb and flow of everyone's clock is a little different, morning larks may want to eat breakfast as their energy levels climb in the morning, whereas night owls might prefer to eat later. An emerging field of science called "chrononutrition" looks at how best to eat according to your chronotype, but research is still at an early stage.

There's no evidence that eating breakfast will make you healthier, and the significance of breakfast is usually down to an individual's preference, lifestyle, and body clock. However, children, the unwell, those with diabetes, and people who do heavy manual work should make breakfast a priority, to provide ready-access fuel for the body and brain, and to avoid burning fat.

Will Skipping Breakfast Make Me Fat?

The good news for breakfast dodgers is that piling on pounds isn't inevitable—as long as you control those high-calorie cravings and stay active.

Research shows that although avoiding breakfast will make you hungrier and you might make up for that with a bigger lunch, this won't necessarily make you "fatter"—on average, those who skip breakfast don't eat more across the whole day than if they didn't skip it. Some researchers have found that you may even eat fewer calories overall and end up using your body's fat reserves for energy, which can actually help you lose weight.

However, weight isn't the only consideration; studies show that

IN ONE STUDY, **DIETERS** WHO **SKIPPED BREAKFAST** OVER 12 WEEKS **LOST** AN AVERAGE OF **4** LB

breakfast skippers are likely to exercise less. This may be because they have lower energy levels—after eight hours or so without food, the body will have used up most of its stores of easy-to-access energy during sleep. Morning fasters are also more likely to have unhealthy but appetite-suppressing habits, such as smoking or drinking a lot of coffee.

If you want to ensure that you eat a regular, nourishing breakfast, try preparing it the night before—don't leave it until the morning, when your brain struggles to make good decisions (see pages 12–13).

IF YOU DO SKIP BREAKFAST...

- **Don't overcompensate** with a uge lunch; otherwise, you'll suffer a post-lunch slump (see pages 102–103).
- **Make sure** you eat something before you exercise, or you risk "hitting the wall" (see page 164).
- **Don't make up for lack of energy** with coffee—it can suppress your appetite and make you jittery.

What's the Best Thing to Eat for Breakfast?

Breakfast isn't the magical meal it's billed to be. But it's your first opportunity to refill the fuel stores after your body's overnight fast, so choose energizing foods.

Most people around the world eat in the morning before they set out for their day. How much we eat varies by culture and cuisine—a cup of instant noodles is a popular grab-and-go food with East Asian commuters, while a croissant or pastry with a cup of coffee is the morning sustenance enjoyed in many European countries.

There are no golden rules for a perfect breakfast, but across cultures, most breakfasts are made up mainly of unrefined carbohydrates, such as brown bread or rice, whole grains, and vegetables, all of which contain starch. This is no coincidence. Starch is the best energy source for your ravenously hungry brain and the optimum fuel for replenishing the body's stores of glycogen that have been depleted overnight. Starches are gradually digested in the intestines and converted into brain-friendly sugars. Fiber in the same food slows the digestion process even further, ensuring a longer-term energy supply.

FEELING HUNGRY?

This graph shows how different foods affect how much and for how long you feel full: unrefined rye will keep you fuller for longer than cornflakes, made from highly refined corn.

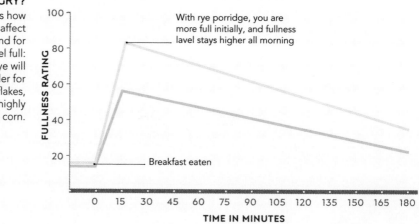

With rye porridge, you are more full initially, and fullness lavel stays higher all morning

Breakfast eaten

FULLNESS RATING

TIME IN MINUTES

KEY
- Rye porridge
- Cornflakes

Be wary—convenient breakfasts often come at a cost. For example, instant porridge and whole grain porridge may look similar and have identical ingredients, but the body handles them quite differently. The rolled oats in instant porridge are sliced small and steamed before packing so that they cook faster, but their starches are part-cooked and the fiber is damaged, meaning they release energy much faster and they won't keep you as full as slower-cooked rolled oats. In one study, teens were given instant or whole grain oats for breakfast; those who ate the quick-cook variety became hungrier much sooner and ended up eating 53 percent more calories at lunch.

Refined starches, such as those found in white bread and rice, not only release their sugars faster than unrefined counterparts, but much of their fiber, nutrients, and minerals are also lost when they are processed.

To add to your starch-based, ideally nonprocessed breakfast, you can eat fresh fruit or vegetables for extra vitamins and fiber, protein to fill you up, and fat to help repair nerves and absorb vitamins. Limit sugary foods, since sugar supplies only short-term energy and is a powerful driver for tooth decay.

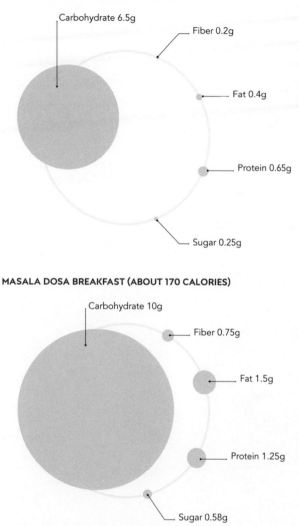

CONGEE BREAKFAST (ABOUT 215 CALORIES)

Carbohydrate 6.5g

Fiber 0.2g

Fat 0.4g

Protein 0.65g

Sugar 0.25g

MASALA DOSA BREAKFAST (ABOUT 170 CALORIES)

Carbohydrate 10g

Fiber 0.75g

Fat 1.5g

Protein 1.25g

Sugar 0.58g

COMPARING BREAKFASTS

Breakfasts vary considerably across the world, and no nation has the "perfect" breakfast. Two typical breakfasts from China and India, respectively, are shown here. Congee is a rice porridge that is particularly energy-rich. Masala dosas are spicy vegan pancakes made with ground rice and lentils.

What's the Healthiest Breakfast Cereal?

Don't be deceived by the images on your cereal box of alpine vistas, ripe fruits, and shiny nuts—what's inside may turn out to be far from wholesome.

The packaging on breakfast cereal brands can be deceiving; words such as "granola" and "natural" are not guarantees that the contents will be health-enhancing. Instead, look at the ingredients and nutrition information, usually given in a table. Most modern-day breakfast cereals contain high amounts of sugar.

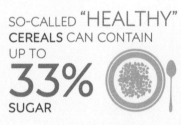

SO-CALLED "HEALTHY" CEREALS CAN CONTAIN UP TO

33%
SUGAR

A CEREAL CONSPIRACY

Breakfast cereals were once tasteless affairs, quite unlike the heavily sweet ones we are used to today. When the entrepreneurial brother of corn flakes' inventor JH Kellogg decided to add sugar to their product, premade cereals became the go-to morning meal for the masses. Since the early 1920s, breakfast cereal makers have gradually increased levels of salt, sugar, and flavorings to tantalize consumers' taste buds.

Avoid highly processed products such as flakes and hoops. The body absorbs these too quickly because the starches are partly broken down during processing.

Aim instead for minimally processed grains, such as porridge, oatmeal, or low-sugar mueslis—these provide a longer-lasting supply of fuel throughout the morning.

Most ready-to-eat breakfast cereals contain a range of added vitamins, minerals, and fiber, which offer a nutritional safety net for picky eaters. This "fortification" is not necessarily an indicator of better or healthier cereals, though—many of these nutrients were in the cereals in the first place but were stripped away during the products' heavy processing. Some synthetic nutrients, such as iron, may not even be absorbed by the body as well as they would have been from the whole food.

Try making your own cereals using fruits, seeds, and nuts.

Is Juicing a Good Way to Get One of My Five a Day?

Breakfast juice is a much-loved tradition that's supposedly healthy and vitamin-packed. Juice does count as one of your five a day, but you're not getting the most out of it.

Ideas that a glass or three of fruit or vegetable juice will cure cancer, wash out "toxins," or even prevent the common cold need squashing for good—all these claims have been comprehensively disproved. Juices can be a convenient way to get a daily dose of vitamins and minerals but are nearly always second best to eating the whole fruit. Juices can be very sugary and acidic and are corrosive to teeth (see page 33).

Smoothies made from the whole, pulverized fruit are better because they retain the gut-friendly fiber. But drink them immediately—many vitamins and antioxidants begin disintegrating from the moment the fruit is sliced.

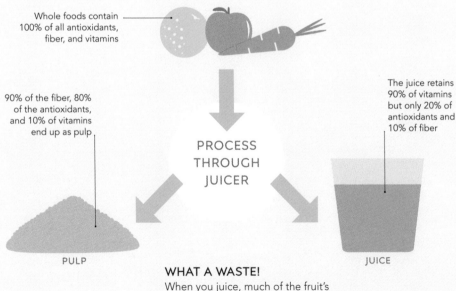

Whole foods contain 100% of all antioxidants, fiber, and vitamins

90% of the fiber, 80% of the antioxidants, and 10% of vitamins end up as pulp

The juice retains 90% of vitamins but only 20% of antioxidants and 10% of fiber

PROCESS THROUGH JUICER

PULP

JUICE

WHAT A WASTE!
When you juice, much of the fruit's goodness goes straight to the pulp bin.

Should I Take Vitamins with My Breakfast?

Logic tells us that if vitamins are good, then a lot more vitamins must be even better—but the science turns out to be a bit more complex than that.

Worried that our food may not be enough to keep us fully healthy, many of us like the convenience of nature's goodness condensed into a tablet. In general, supplements are harmless but often unnecessary. Research shows that people who take supplements are on average more health-conscious and already eat a balanced diet.

Also, some vitamins can't easily be absorbed on their own—if you don't

67%
OF **AMERICANS** SAY THEY REGULARLY TAKE A **MULTIVITAMIN** SUPPLEMENT

take them with the right foods, your good intentions (and money) will be flushed down the toilet.

In certain cases, supplements have saved millions of lives and improved the well-being of countless more. Across the globe, iron tablets are used to reverse anemia, folic acid (vitamin B9) prevents spinal deformities developing in newborns, and vitamin A helps prevent blindness and life-threatening immune system deficiencies.

Some vitamins are also antioxidants because they neutralize free radicals—toxic waste substances that are continuously created within your body as part of normal daily wear and tear. Logic would suggest that taking even more antioxidants would give you a helping hand. Surprisingly, the

THE SPREAD OF "VITAMIN MANIA"

The modern-day vitamin craze can be traced back to the scientist Linus Pauling, who, having already won two Nobel Prizes, was aiming for a third. In the 1970s, he claimed that taking huge doses of vitamin C—found in citrus fruits and many vegetables—would eradicate the common cold, fight cancer, and avert heart disease. The outspoken researcher's impossible claims started "vitamin mania"—and even though his research has been thoroughly debunked, we have never looked back.

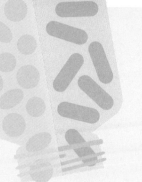

OIL-SOLUBLE VITAMINS

Taken as multivitamin supplements, these vitamins will still be absorbed by the body but won't be absorbed as optimally as if they were eaten with or in certain foods.

WATER-SOLUBLE VITAMINS

These vitamins can't be stored in the body. If you take a supplement when you already have enough, the body simply flushes it away in your urine.

Vitamin A: essential for healthy vision and helps growth; found in leafy greens, liver, and fish oil

A

C

Vitamin C: antioxidant and helps tissues repair; found in many fruits and vegetables

Vitamin D: helps the body absorb calcium; found in oily fish and created in skin with sunlight

D

B2

Vitamin B2 (riboflavin): helps the body release energy from food; important for growth. Found in meat, milk, and rice

Vitamin E: antioxidant, boosts the immune system; found in avocados, nuts, and olive oil

E

B9

Vitamin B9 (folic acid): helps produce new cells. Essential in pregnancy. Found in chickpeas, broccoli, and bananas

Vitamin K: allows blood to clot well, helping wounds heal; found in leafy greens and cereal

K

B12

MULTIVITAMIN TABLETS

Vitamin B12: used to make blood cells and helps nerves function properly; found in meat and eggs

opposite is sometimes true. Free radicals are also generated after exercise, and they alert your body to repair and rebuild. Experiments have shown that excessive levels of the antioxidant vitamins C and E mop up these free radicals too quickly for your body to detect, which means that the repair process is impaired. Just as you need exercise to keep everything running smoothly, it seems that the body's defense systems need a molecular workout to stay fighting fit. Studies have also shown that too many antioxidants can even accelerate the spread of some cancers. This is because malignant cells also release free radicals, and if these are swept away before the body's defenses are alerted, it's then easier for cancer cells to multiply under the cloak of seemingly protective antioxidants.

Most of us, unless we have a medical need, can get all the vitamins and minerals we require from a balanced, varied diet. Taking supplements almost certainly won't give you a long life—but eating well just might.

It's Cold! Should I Wear a Thick Sweater or Layers?

When it's cold, the trick to staying warm is to pick clothes with different thicknesses that will create a cozy bubble of insulating, warm air around your body.

The clothes that keep us toasty do so because they trap a cushion of air around us that is warmed up by the body. It's the air, rather than the fabric itself, that keeps us warm, so think twice before splurging on high-tech clothing. As strange as it sounds, stagnant air is better than almost anything else at retaining heat—that's why there is a gap between the panes of double-pane windows.

It's not the number of layers or the thickness of the material that is most important; the key is to create the biggest, most stable, blanket of air all around your body that won't be blown away by the wind. This is why baggy T-shirts and flowing pullovers are no good, even if you wear lots of them.

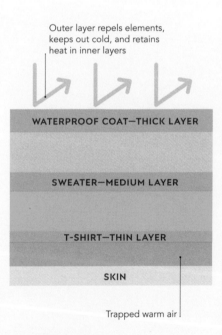

Outer layer repels elements, keeps out cold, and retains heat in inner layers

WATERPROOF COAT—THICK LAYER

SWEATER—MEDIUM LAYER

T-SHIRT—THIN LAYER

SKIN

Trapped warm air

BRACING YOURSELF FOR THE CHILLY OUTDOORS?

1

WEAR WOOL OR SYNTHETIC FUR because they trap lots of air between their fibers, which forms another layer of insulation around your body.

2

LAYER UP with a well-fitting thin layer close to your skin to lock in air, covered by one or two looser, thicker layers.

LAYERING UP

The best way to keep out extreme cold is to wear a thin layer next to the skin, followed by two progressively thicker layers, to trap maximum air.

It's Hot! What Should I Wear to Keep Cool?

Sweating is the body's go-to climate control and is the key to avoiding overheating. It's important to wear clothes that allow sweat to evaporate easily.

When it's hot enough to fry an egg on the pavement, the stream of salty sweat that drips from your skin is your life-saving lotion—by evaporating off your skin, sweat removes heat from your body, cooling you down. The more skin that is exposed to air, the faster sweat can turn to vapor.

Loose clothing or bare skin lets your body heat radiate out directly—avoid thick, clinging clothing on a hot day, which will stop your sweat from evaporating and keep your skin damp and hot. It's important to wear sunscreen to protect completely exposed skin, but beware that some creams can slow sweat production, making you hotter.

Dark colors absorb heat, so aren't good for hot weather. Oddly though, the desert-dwelling Bedouin people famously wear black robes. Research has revealed that although the outside of their garments becomes ferociously hot, the fabric is so thick and loose-fitting that the heat doesn't make it through and the shielded skin stays relatively cool.

Some specialty clothing is made from fabrics that can wick (pull) sweat away from the skin through microscopic gaps between fibers, to help the body better regulate its temperature. Some advanced fabrics are made of materials or beads that swell when moistened by sweat, absorbing heat as they expand.

A NEW **PLASTIC-BASED FABRIC** CAN KEEP SKIN AROUND **4°F COOLER** THAN **COTTON**

WANT TO **STAY COOL** ON A **HOT DAY?**

1

WEAR LOOSE COTTON OR LINEN CLOTHING so that air can flow over your skin, speeding up sweat evaporation.

2

WEAR LIGHT COLORS to minimize the heat your clothes absorb.

3

WEAR CLOTHES MADE OF WICKING FIBERS such as nylon, polyester, or polypropylene if exercising or sweating.

Do We Burn More Calories When It's Colder?

By turning down the thermostat, some people say that you can shed the pounds. Surprisingly, science agrees that it should work, but just don't expect fast results.

When the temperature dives, patches of brown fat scattered around your body (see page 46) burn like miniature furnaces, cranking up your internal temperature and burning calories in the process. You'll burn an extra 80–100 calories if you turn the thermostat down from a comfy 72°F (22°C) to a cool 64°F (18°C) over the course of a morning. Persisting with this strategy

every morning for a year would, in theory, net you nearly 11 lb (5 kg) in lost weight! No long-term studies prove or disprove the idea, but it is a promising theory. However, the bad news is that when it's cold, your primal instincts tell you to eat more to lay down layers of insulating fat; most people eat more than enough to offset any weight-loss effects of cooler temperatures.

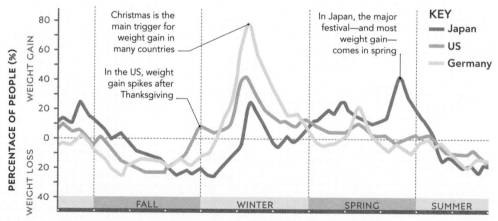

CALORIFIC CELEBRATIONS
This 2016 study shows that, where winter coincides with major festivities, it's actually the season of weight gain, not loss.

" **Shivering** not only spurs your **active muscle tissue to** generate **heat** but also releases a hormone that **triggers brown fat cells** into action. "

Is Central Heating Bad for Our Health?

Unless you're used to braving colder climates, the way your body regulates its own temperature has become sluggish, and central heating may be to blame.

Centrally heated homes and a room-temperature world has led us to lose a natural type of heat-generating fat called brown fat—you emerge from the womb with plenty of it, but as you age and you don't use it, this brown fat withers away. When you're cold, brown fat (controlled by nerves connected to the brain) heats the body rapidly by sucking energy out of the normal white fat that clings unhealthily to your organs and under your skin. This process also burns lots of calories, boosting your metabolism. By rendering brown fat unnecessary, central heating, in the long run, can be unhealthy.

CENTRAL HEATING
REDUCES **BROWN FAT**, WHICH PLAYS A KEY ROLE IN PREVENTING OBESITY

It's possible to reverse this loss by braving the cold once more. Research shows that regular doses of cold weather or dips in icy cold water—especially when combined with exercise—stimulate brown fat patches to regrow, making you better at handling the cold. So try turning down the thermostat once in a while, because with more of these small fat-burning furnaces dotted around the body, you might be able to lose those love handles a little faster.

KEY
White fat
Brown fat

PERSONAL FURNACES
We have less brown fat than white fat, although women have more than men. Brown fat is mostly found in small patches on the upper body.

Is Air-Conditioning Unhealthy, Too?

Air-conditioning is essential in many industries, such as computer hardware and textiles, but are we exchanging commodities and comfort for our health?

Air-conditioning has a lot going for it. AC units filter out air and particle pollution (partly why you are less likely to die from a heart attack if your home or workplace is air-conditioned). It's also great for productivity; quality of work improves in comfortable temperatures, allergies are often less bothersome, and the risk of heat stroke is reduced in hot countries.

However, many people are worried that the humming box could be making them sick—and sickness rates are, in fact, higher in workplaces with AC. AC strips moisture from the air and so can dry out the air and exacerbate existing conditions such as eczema. Neglected units can accumulate mold, dust, and microbes, potentially spreading invisible nasties and illnesses such as Legionnaires' disease, so it's important to keep AC systems clean and serviced.

Stopping short of cleaning the office AC yourself, you can moisturize to keep your skin healthy, and take regular walks outside to limit time spent with the AC.

Do Women Really Feel the Cold More Than Men?

The war over the home and office thermostat will never end. Everyone has their own preferred temperature, but can the battle lines really be drawn between the sexes?

Women really do hate the cold more. Not because men are especially miserly about heating costs or that females are weaker or have a lower threshold for discomfort. Rather, biology is at play in this quarrel Men are generally better equipped to deal with cold than women, owing to their larger size and more heat-producing muscle bulk. Women appear to be programmed to feel the cold: in an identically proportioned and muscled man and woman, the woman would have slightly colder fingers and toes. This is partly because women have higher levels of estrogen—a hormone that thickens their blood, reducing warming blood flow to the outer parts of the body.

Women have a range of biological tics, too: cold-sensing nerves in their skin detect a temperature drop faster than men, their skin pales quicker as blood is diverted away to reduce heat loss, and they shiver sooner at higher temperatures than men do. We don't know exactly why these differences exist, but some scientists think that women are better evolved to hold on to their body heat, diverting it from the skin inward, to where a growing child may be.

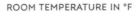

ROOM TEMPERATURE IN °F

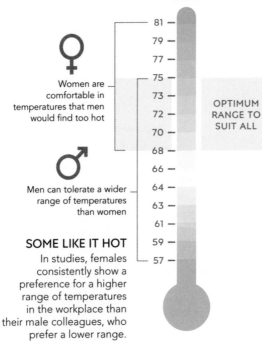

Women are comfortable in temperatures that men would find too hot

81
79
77
75
73
72
70
68

OPTIMUM RANGE TO SUIT ALL

Men can tolerate a wider range of temperatures than women

66
64
63
61
59
57

SOME LIKE IT HOT

In studies, females consistently show a preference for a higher range of temperatures in the workplace than their male colleagues, who prefer a lower range.

" Temperature tolerance is a **sex divide** that's not imagined—in shared spaces, a **compromise** is the only way to **keep the peace**. "

Will Wearing a Coat Indoors Mean I'm Colder When I Go Out?

We're told that wrapping up before going outside means "you won't feel the full benefit," but this apparent wisdom leaves scientists cold.

Wearing a coat indoors for several minutes before stepping outside will mean you may not "feel" the benefit in the form of an instant hit of relief from the cold, but you will definitely be getting it. Day and night, your body relentlessly churns out heat, so wearing a sturdy outdoor coat before stepping outside is a good start because it traps this heat around your body. When you go outside with your coat on, you may not feel the sudden change of temperature around your chest, because you'll have already surrounded yourself in a comfy bubble of body-warmed air (see page 42)—but you're definitely still reaping the benefit.

THE HEAT THAT **YOUR BODY PUMPS OUT** IS EQUIVALENT TO A

100w

TUNGSTEN LIGHT BULB

As you get older and your skin becomes wrinkled, the temperature sensors in the skin wither away, and you don't feel the cold as strongly—this is why the elderly are at a higher risk of hypothermia, so layering up before you begin to feel cold is particularly important for older people. Also, if you're unwell or have heart problems, layer up before you go out to minimize any strain on the heart and circulatory system from the sudden plunge in temperature.

That said, if your coat is making you too warm, then that's not a good thing. You certainly don't want to have a flushed face and damp skin when you step outside. Sweating will make your exposed skin considerably colder than it would have been.

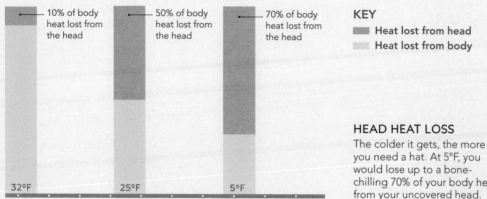

10% of body heat lost from the head

50% of body heat lost from the head

70% of body heat lost from the head

KEY
Heat lost from head
Heat lost from body

32°F   25°F   5°F

OUTSIDE TEMPERATURE

HEAD HEAT LOSS
The colder it gets, the more you need a hat. At 5°F, you would lose up to a bone-chilling 70% of your body heat from your uncovered head.

Do I Lose Most of My Body Heat from My Head?

Covering your head on a cold day is a no-brainer—but if you had to choose between wearing a hat or pants, it's clear that this scientific-sounding saying is off the mark.

This health tidbit taught by parents everywhere seems to have originally come from the 1957 edition of the US Army Survival Guide. The military manual said that "40 to 45 percent of body heat" escapes through the head, although the original meaning has been taken out of context.

On a cold day, your head radiates heat out like a lantern, but this escaping warmth doesn't add up to "40 to 45 percent" of your body's heat loss—let alone most of it. When you're naked, only about 10 percent of

heat made by the body radiates from the head—far more is lost from the larger surfaces of the torso, arms, and legs. Only if the temperature is very low, and you are wearing thick insulated gear everywhere else, would the Army Manual apply—it described soldiers who were without hat or ear muffs but otherwise well wrapped up.

So Mom was right—but only if it's colder than 25°F and you are already wrapped up in good cold-weather clothing but foolish enough to not be wearing a hat.

Is Commuting Harming My Health?

About 4 billion of us travel between home and work, school, or college. Is our daily commute just something we love to hate or a major health hazard?

Some form of commuting has been a part of our lives since the Neolithic age, and although we love to complain about our commutes, research shows that we wouldn't want it any other way. We're generally happiest when we have at least some distance between where we sleep and relax and where we spend the bulk of our day. However, there are limits. We view our commute as part of our job, and if the trip length makes us unhappy, we're more likely to quit—so much so that an extra 20 minutes' commuting time can reduce job satisfaction by the same amount as a 20 percent pay cut.

Length of trip is the major factor in commuting: in the morning, your body clock is winding up the brain and body—alertness and attention increases with each passing minute, and if you're stuck in traffic or a broken-down train during this precious prime time, then the most productive part of your day could be lost in transit. A morning commute of 45 minutes or more seems to be the tipping point at which the trip length starts to take a toll on physical and mental health. Workers who travel more than 90 minutes each day are less fit, weigh more, and have higher blood pressure, compared to those with a shorter travel time. Longer commutes are also linked to health issues such as sleep problems, exhaustion, aches and pains, and overeating. Moreover,

WANT TO IMPROVE YOUR COMMUTE?

1

WALK, JOG, OR CYCLE—moving under your own power releases mood-lifting hormones and increases blood flow to the brain, making you happier and more productive.

2

SIMPLIFY TRIPS that involve more than one stop, for example, taking children to school on the way to work. Multiple-stage trips are the most stressful.

3

PLAN YOUR DAY and spend the time mentally adjusting to work mode on the way in, and winding down on the commute home.

4

FIND A NEW JOB if your commute is more than 90 minutes long—your health is probably suffering!

unpredictable and stressful delays, the chances of which increase the longer your commute, make the biggest negative impact on your health.

The method of travel also plays a part in how healthy your commute is. Driving takes the cake as the most stressful and unhealthiest way to commute. Public transportation always comes out better, but simply using your legs to get to work—be it by walking, cycling, or jogging—beats both.

Scientists have shown that a "good" commute is one that is long enough to

15 MINUTES
IS THE OPTIMUM LENGTH OF TIME FOR A COMMUTE

give us time to draw a psychological line between home life and work but not so long that it makes us anxious, bored, or tired. Even if you work from home, you can benefit from a "virtual" commute by going for a short walk, run, or cycle to mark the start and end of your working day.

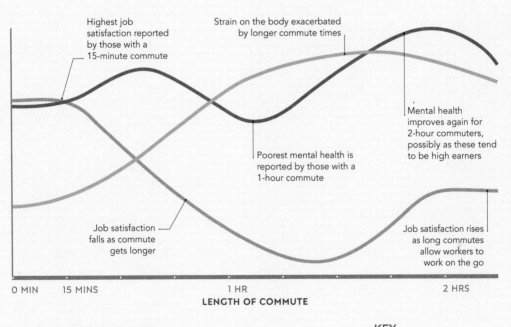

Highest job satisfaction reported by those with a 15-minute commute

Strain on the body exacerbated by longer commute times

Poorest mental health is reported by those with a 1-hour commute

Mental health improves again for 2-hour commuters, possibly as these tend to be high earners

Job satisfaction falls as commute gets longer

Job satisfaction rises as long commutes allow workers to work on the go

0 MIN   15 MINS   1 HR   2 HRS
LENGTH OF COMMUTE

EFFECTS OF COMMUTING
Studies show that our mental and physical health and job satisfaction are closely connected with the length of our daily commute.

KEY
▬ Job satisfaction
▬ Mental health
▬ Physical strain

Why Does My Morning Commute Seem Longer?

When traveling or commuting—be it by car, train, or bike—
we go through a strange time warp with the trip there
feeling longer than the trip back.

Our brains are unreliable stopwatches, unconsciously piecing together clues to "guesstimate" the passage of time. Familiar sights and sounds are deemed unworthy of wasting precious brain power over, so humdrum routes such as daily commutes generally get squashed in our memory banks and feel shorter than they really are.

On the other hand, the very first trip to somewhere new will feel much longer than the same trip taken at a later time, simply because new experiences are remembered better—which is why children often complain ("Are we there yet?") when stuck in the back seat of a long car trip but rarely say a peep on the way back. However,

OUR **MORNING TRIP** TO WORK **FEELS** AS THOUGH IT'S **AROUND** 20% **LONGER** THAN IT ACTUALLY IS

your expectations of the trip and unexpected stress play a part in this time warp, too. When you're late for work and fighting for a space on the train, your brain is awash with adrenaline and other fight-or-flight chemicals. This sudden anxiety and stress, coupled with the natural morning flood of energizing cortisol (see page 15), puts the brakes on time by making the brain fire faster—so your morning commute will always seem longer than your evening one. Also, your memory circuitry soaks up these stressful experiences like a sponge. Once you do make it into work and find yourself retelling the stressful experience, this will only embed the ordeal into long-term memory, adding to the trip's significance and perceived length.

This evolved instinct to ruminate over events that have threatened us in the past has helped humankind learn how to avoid hungry predators and, these days, dodge the badly driven bus. You can't escape this time warp, even when it comes to uneventful trips—

anything that brings the passing of time to the forefront of our awareness will make your travel time feel longer. Clock-watching is also a sure-fire way to make a slow morning commute drag. Try distracting yourself from checking the minute hand by listening to an interesting podcast or uplifting music. This will occupy your mind and make memories of the traveling hazier. Who knows, it might even make your endless morning commute fun!

LET'S DO THE TIME WARP

This study shows just how bad we are at estimating how long our trips take: the shorter the trip, the more likely we are to overestimate its duration.

KEY

■ Reported trip time longer than actual trip time

▨ Reported trip time shorter than actual trip time

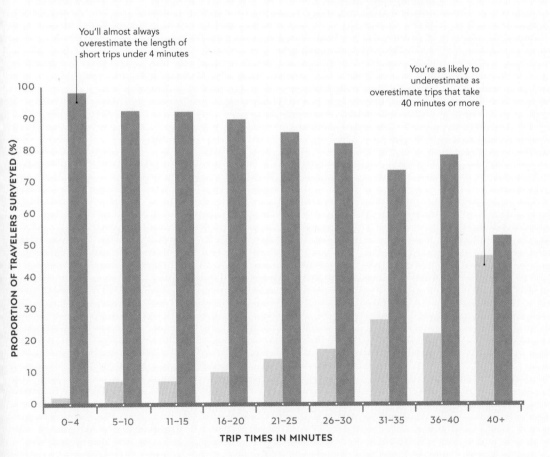

You'll almost always overestimate the length of short trips under 4 minutes

You're as likely to underestimate as overestimate trips that take 40 minutes or more

PROPORTION OF TRAVELERS SURVEYED (%)

TRIP TIMES IN MINUTES

Why Are People in Cities So Rude?

If you need help in a city, the more people there are around, the less likely it is that anyone will come to your aid. Are city dwellers callous, or is there something else going on?

Lack of helpfulness in the city is a real phenomenon; nearly everyone would help someone in need if they were alone, while few would come forward if in a large group of strangers.

It's a perverse part of human nature: when we're in a large crowd, a herd instinct kicks in and we naturally assume that someone else will step in—a phenomenon known as "diffusion of responsibility." A positive step can be infectious, though—tin-rattling charity collectors are ignored until someone is seen to donate, after which other would-be givers imitate and come forward. Try being brave: make a positive gesture, and you may influence others to do the same.

Town planners also share some of the blame for the briskness of city dwellers. By simply adding a few more shrubs and signposts, a city can be made more compassionate. On featureless streets, lined by drab concrete, metal walls, or large panes of glass, pedestrians walk quickly and look straight ahead. However, studies show that on roads with plants, colored walls, and uneven surfaces (termed an "active edge"), the average pace of walkers is slower: people tend to glance around more and feel less anxious. Incredibly enough, just a small drop in walking speed has been linked to increasing the chances that someone will start up conversation and help out a stranger in need.

If you like city life but find yourself disheartened by all the unfriendliness, consider living in neighborhoods full of colors and greenery. You could even get involved in your local area or community and spruce up your neighborhood by planting more trees or decorating with artwork and other colorful features.

5% OF A CROWD
CAN **CONTROL** THE
MOVEMENTS OF **THE REST**

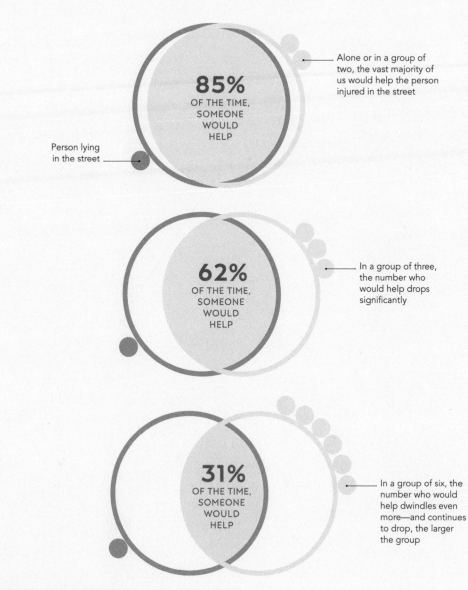

Alone or in a group of two, the vast majority of us would help the person injured in the street

85% OF THE TIME, SOMEONE WOULD HELP

Person lying in the street

In a group of three, the number who would help drops significantly

62% OF THE TIME, SOMEONE WOULD HELP

In a group of six, the number who would help dwindles even more—and continues to drop, the larger the group

31% OF THE TIME, SOMEONE WOULD HELP

THE BYSTANDER EFFECT

Our apparent callousness toward a person in need is termed the "bystander effect." When someone is unconscious in the street, most passersby won't trust their instincts to help but look to how others react. If everyone else looks calm, we think there is no emergency. No one helps because no one is helping.

Is Life Really Faster-Paced in the City?

Amidst constant traffic and an army of commuters, it can seem as if city life hurtles at breakneck speed. You aren't imagining it; it really is fast-paced—and it's getting faster.

Since the 1970s, watchful researchers have charted the speed of pedestrians in towns and cities across the globe. Their findings confirm their hunch that the bigger and richer the metropolis, the faster everyone dashes around.

But why are city dwellers in such a rush, anyway? One theory is that larger, wealthier cities have higher rates of pay, meaning there is more worker competition and greater motive to get to work early. The "time is money" philosophy makes the stakes of a missed appointment that much higher.

A simpler and more credible reason surfaced when researchers looked at who actually lives in cities. It seems that the faster pace is simply because more young people are in the centers of the largest, richest cities, Sky-high property prices and tall apartment buildings aren't attractive to the elderly and differently abled. Crowds of competitive youngsters' legs move quickly, making the rest of us feel like we're living in the slow lane.

CITY SLICKERS
The larger the city, the faster people tend to walk. On average, urbanites in the city-state Singapore walk around 30% faster than the residents of Ottawa, which has only one-quarter of Singapore's population.

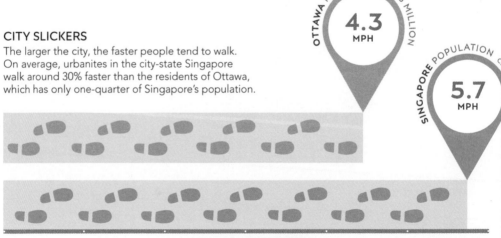

OTTAWA POPULATION c.1.3 MILLION
4.3 MPH

SINGAPORE POPULATION c.5...
5.7 MPH

AVERAGE WALKING SPEED

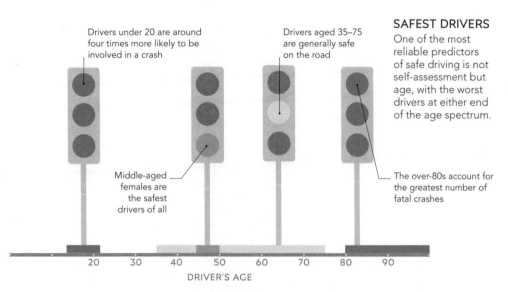

Drivers under 20 are around four times more likely to be involved in a crash

Drivers aged 35–75 are generally safe on the road

SAFEST DRIVERS
One of the most reliable predictors of safe driving is not self-assessment but age, with the worst drivers at either end of the age spectrum.

Middle-aged females are the safest drivers of all

The over-80s account for the greatest number of fatal crashes

DRIVER'S AGE

Why Is Everyone Worse at Driving Than Me?

You're almost certainly not as good a driver as you think. When asked, most drivers rate themselves as "above average"—a mathematical impossibility!

We are all inclined to think so many substandard drivers are hogging the streets because we suffer the human curse of exaggerating our own abilities—this is the Dunning-Kruger effect. It's a mental quirk that clouds almost every area of our lives, although it was probably useful for emboldening our ancestors to be brave instead of cowering in a cave.

In tests, most people think they have performed better than they really did.

The poorer our abilities, the more blissfully ignorant we are of the fact. Conversely, research shows that only the top experts judge themselves too harshly.

No one is immune to the Dunning-Kruger effect, and the only way to gain a realistic insight into your skills is to be independently assessed. Why not take an advanced driving course and find out whether the other drivers really are as inept as you think?

Why Do I Get Road Rage When I'm Normally Calm?

The unique nature of driving—being isolated in a metal shell—alters our mindset and makes us prone to make unfair assumptions, rash judgments, and worse.

On your morning commute, a taxi cuts in without warning, or a student driver stalls at the traffic lights. There's a good chance that, along with most other drivers, these motoring mishaps would have you honking your horn, shaking your fist, or turning the air blue with profanities.

So what causes you to get so uncharacteristically furious? Walled off from everyone else, you can't see other drivers' body language properly or hear them if they mumble an apology, so you're more likely to make unfair assumptions ("They're such a bad driver!"). A crooked thinking process called "fundamental attribution error" means that we excuse our own blunders as being beyond our control, but we judge others' actions much more harshly; for example, you might assume a driver is simply incompetent and inconsiderate rather than possibly being distracted by a screaming child in the back seat.

To top it off, the anonymous sound-proofed world inside your car means that there are fewer constraints to keep a lid on spiraling anger. You can behave in ways that would be unimaginable had the same offending person bumped into you in the street.

In addition to these psychological responses, a biological reaction occurs, too—anything that impedes our haste to get from A to B will fire up a primitive fight-or-flight response. Adrenaline seeps into the blood: heart rate accelerates, blood pressure climbs, muscles get tense, and your thinking

HOW CAN I **CALM THE BEAST** WITHIN?

1

LEAVE IN PLENTY OF TIME to allow for delays; it's when plans are thwarted that you're more likely to lose the plot.

2

PLAY RELAXING MUSIC to counteract the effect of fight-or-flight responses. However, loud, fast music will ramp up feelings of rage.

3

KEEP PHOTOS OF LOVED ONES VISIBLE—this activates the frontal, thinking parts of the brain, helping you retain a sense of empathy.

becomes narrowed and focused. The prefrontal cortex in your brain usually sends powerful calming signals that halt impulsive behavior, but when blood is awash with fight-or-flight hormones, these soothing messages are dialed down. Much of the sensible frontal lobe circuitry that houses your calm personality and good nature becomes disengaged, causing us to become blind to everything other than the threat before us. While it's a useful biological response for protecting yourself from a predator, it's a total

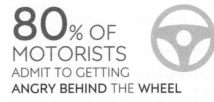

80% OF MOTORISTS
ADMIT TO GETTING
ANGRY BEHIND THE WHEEL

overreaction when trying to navigate through busy traffic.

If driving brings out the uglier side of you, take heart: you're not a passenger when it comes to your emotions and you can regain control of yourself (see pages 62–63).

49% DISTRACTED BY ANOTHER DRIVER

16% DRIVING IN THE CITY

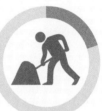

20% CONSTRUCTION

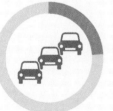

24% HEAVY TRAFFIC

16% WERE HAVING A BAD DAY

39% AGGRESSIVE DRIVERS

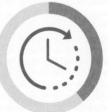

39% RUNNING LATE

EXCUSES, EXCUSES
Drivers who experience road rage cite a number of reasons why they blew their lid. These percentages represent the proportion of people polled who gave that cause as a reason for their rage.

How Can I Shake Off a Bad Mood?

We trust our emotions, believing that they tell us something true about the world, but they are actually a creation of our mind, over which we have a surprising amount of control.

On your way into work on a packed train, somebody shoves you and you drop your phone, and they don't apologize—how rude! You're a little peeved and may have a short fuse for the rest of the morning.

However, emotions aren't something that happen to you because of forces out of your control, rolling in like weather from the sea. Rather, the rich palette of your emotional life is crafted in your mind, directed by the

sensations within your body in response to what you think is happening around you, and also by your past experiences.

This little-known sense, called "interoception," is your mind's sense of what is happening in your body. Like an inward-looking eye, your brain continually surveys the landscape of your internal organs and tissues. To build a picture, the brain files these countless sensations—only some

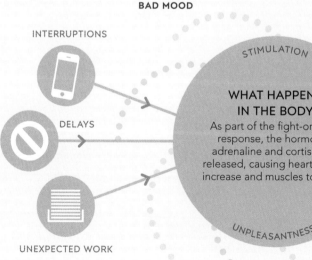

BAD MOOD

INTERRUPTIONS

DELAYS

UNEXPECTED WORK

STIMULATION

WHAT HAPPENS IN THE BODY
As part of the fight-or-flight response, the hormones adrenaline and cortisol are released, causing heart rate to increase and muscles to tense.

INTERPRETED INTO A MOOD/ EMOTION

UNPLEASANTNESS

of which we are consciously aware of—into degrees of four primal states of pleasantness, unpleasantness, calmness, and stimulation. From these states, a blurry image is formed from which mood and emotion are birthed as the brain tries to make sense of what's going on. Studies have shown that when people are injected with a drug that makes the heart race and blood pressure climb, they spontaneously start to feel threatened and angry. The brain simply picks up on bodily sensations to form the basis for our emotions.

When it comes to being shoved on the train, your body will unconsciously and instantly react with a fight-or-flight response and release testosterone into the bloodstream—you can't avoid that—but you can choose whether or not you turn that into anger. Emotions are a two-way street: you have it in your power to consciously affect and even change your mood.

HOW TO **SHAKE OFF** THAT **DARK CLOUD**

1
GO FOR A POWER WALK because a short burst of exercise can give you a feel-good hit from endorphin pulses (see page 157).

2
TALK TO SOMEBODY—it's a dopamine-fueled tonic to a downbeat spirit. Note that texting does not give you the same emotional nourishment!

3
MAKE SOMETHING with your hands. This lifts your mood by boosting feel-good hormones dopamine and serotonin to a far greater degree than any digital pastimes.

GOOD MOOD

EXERCISE

CALMNESS

BEING SOCIAL

WHAT HAPPENS IN THE BODY
The feel-good hormones serotonin and dopamine are released in the brain and also in the gut. They stabilize heart rate, which helps induce calm.

BEING CREATIVE

PLEASANTNESS

How Can I Get the Most from My Working Day?

If you start the day by checking emails, you're doing it all wrong and risk wasting the brain's golden hours. You're better off tackling challenging tasks in the morning.

For most of us, the morning is when our brains are optimized to solve problems, ignore distractions, and focus on the task at hand; it's unwise to fritter away this prime time by painstakingly deleting spam, writing lengthy email replies, or getting embroiled in a vortex of social media updates. Your boss isn't calling the shots—your body clock is. Lengthy meetings in the morning squander most people's top-speed thinking power, so if you can, shift those commitments away from these premium hours. However, if you're a night owl, bear in mind this mental peak will come in the afternoon.

For most, the morning is the best time for the jobs that need your focused concentration, such as working on a project's budget, planning a multiple-month schedule, or writing a detailed report, or for activities that

The mind is geared up and ready to go—now's the time to take on that challenging task you've been putting off for weeks

OPTIMAL DAY
Your body clock determines when you wake, when you're alert, when you're ready for exercise, and when you're sleepy. Whatever your line of work, you'll be more productive if you work in harmony with your natural internal rhythm.

6:00 AM

10:00 AM

The "thinking" regions of your brain are still waking up this early in the morning, so don't jump straight into challenging tasks

64

require your full attention and quick reactions, such as operating industrial machinery. Try to optimize your workspace (see pages 66–67), and be aware that distractions, such as pop-up

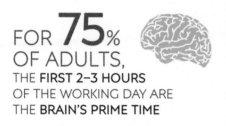

FOR **75**%
OF ADULTS,
THE **FIRST 2–3 HOURS**
OF THE WORKING DAY ARE
THE **BRAIN'S PRIME TIME**

notifications and unexpected phone calls, are a leech on productivity. If you can fit in some light exercise before work, this typically enhances your motivation, concentration, and even academic performance.

By the time lunchtime looms, the end credits on top productivity are starting to roll and you can't rewind this concentration-high with coffee or food. Mundane paperwork, routine meetings, conference calls, and beanbag breaks for bouncing new ideas around with colleagues are best saved for the later parts of the working day when the brain is in "free-thought" mode (see page 70) and the mind is less focused and more relaxed.

Your physical prowess runs a little behind your brain—your heart, lungs, and muscles work best in the afternoon, so it's better to save your most physically demanding tasks until then (see page 150).

As the brain winds down, networks between different regions are more likely to light up, creating "light-bulb" moments, even when you're not thinking of work!

2:30 PM	7:30 PM	10:00 PM

Unless you're a late riser, your muscles have built up steam and your body is primed for physical work

Adenosine levels in the brain are high, making you feel mentally fatigued and your thinking slow and sluggish.

65

What's the Best Workspace for Productivity?

The ideal workspace will encourage both concentration and creative sharing of ideas, and there are plenty of things you can do to achieve these goals.

Whether you work in an office, at home, or in any other environment, your personal workspace is key. Chaos is uncomfortable, but sterile, impersonal, super-neat spaces are actually worse—research shows they stifle creativity and productivity, increase anxiety, and up the risk of Sick Building Syndrome symptoms (see page 74). People perform better in an environment they can customize and make more personal.

However, a degree of tidiness is beneficial. Some studies have shown that a neat and ordered desk aligns your mind to think logically, making you more likely to take measured, sensible decisions, and even make healthier choices—in one study, people who worked in a disorganized workspace (as opposed to a tidy one) were three times more likely to pick a chocolate bar over an apple when offered a snack.

Now think about what's nearby. Noisy workplaces are hard to concentrate in, but complete silence can stifle thought for many. In fact, some background noise, be it the tick of a clock, distant chatter, or musical murmurings from the radio seem to activate the

IDEAL WORKSPACE
You'll want a blend of concentration-meets-comfort: somewhere to put your head down and crack on but also somewhere to put your feet up. Personalized is always better—you'll be more at ease around familiar items.

A relaxing "third space" provides an unpressured area to unwind and reflect on ideas

Ample natural light will boost mood and increase positivity

"watching" brain network and help us stay focused. Around 50 decibels, the sound of rainfall, seems to be the sweet spot for most of us. Extroverted people tend to thrive in noisier places, whereas more reflective types may founder in such an environment. Noise-canceling headphones can be useful—although the downside is you may lose out on valuable interaction with colleagues. In a shared workspace, decisions about noise and tidiness levels invariably require compromise.

If you have the freedom of choosing where and when to work, place yourself somewhere that will help you achieve your specific aim. Need to crack on with that report? Open-plan workspaces are bad for concentration because of distractions, so choose somewhere that minimizes the risk of your attention being disrupted, like a private (preferably personalized!) cubby, and get to work in the morning (see pages 64–65). Need to think out of the box and collaborate with others? Try gathering in pleasant gardens or comfy sofas near a smoothie bar in the afternoon. These informal meeting spots are dubbed the "third space" by architects and are designed to give workers unpressured space to unwind, reflect, and chat through ideas.

PRODUCTIVITY INCREASES
BY 30% WHEN PEOPLE ARE ABLE TO **PERSONALIZE** THEIR **WORKSPACE**

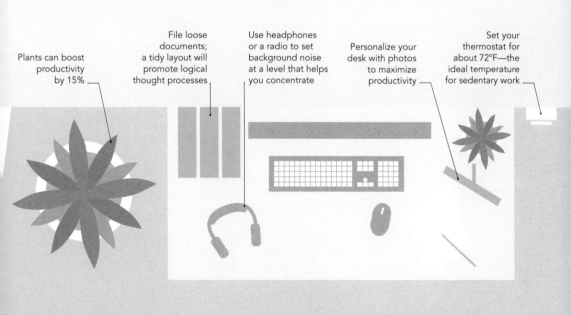

Plants can boost productivity by 15%

File loose documents; a tidy layout will promote logical thought processes

Use headphones or a radio to set background noise at a level that helps you concentrate

Personalize your desk with photos to maximize productivity

Set your thermostat for about 72°F—the ideal temperature for sedentary work

Can I Learn to Be Better at Multitasking?

It's time to nail this myth once and for all—the scientific fact is that your brain is simply not wired for multitasking.

We make the mistake of thinking that our gray matter is like a computer—but try as we may, our conscious thinking powers cannot be split along separate paths in the way that a computer can run multiple programs simultaneously.

It takes between a few milliseconds to several minutes for the brain to fully orient to a new task, depending on the task's complexity. When we dart like a butterfly between tasks, the vast majority of us end up not doing any of them well—we make more mistakes and become less able to remember new things. By continually switching focus—and maybe buzzing on stress-induced adrenaline—we can be blind to how unproductive we're being. Here's the kicker: those who think they're experts at multitasking are actually the worst at it, thanks to the Dunning-Kruger effect (see page 59).

To work with, not against, your brain, prioritize tasks so you know what needs to get done first, cut those email notifications, and avoid starting a job until you've prepared what you need to complete it.

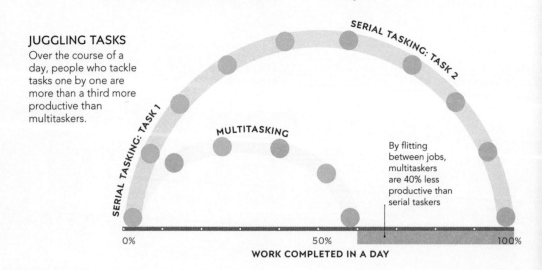

JUGGLING TASKS
Over the course of a day, people who tackle tasks one by one are more than a third more productive than multitaskers.

SERIAL TASKING: TASK 1

SERIAL TASKING: TASK 2

MULTITASKING

By flitting between jobs, multitaskers are 40% less productive than serial taskers

0%   50%   100%

WORK COMPLETED IN A DAY

A plucky 2.5 percent of us take multitasking to the next level; these supertaskers are able to be in charge of a hospital Emergency Department, and not be fazed by a ward full of patients in pain, a crowd of relatives clamoring for attention, and another ambulance due to arrive in the next five minutes.

Somehow, the decision-making cabling in the supertasker's brain is able to fire with great efficiency—doing more work with less effort. Supertaskers can filter out unwanted distractions, remember details easily, and stay as cool as a cucumber when under pressure.

You might wish that you were one of this elite breed, but it seems to be impossible to learn these skills—being a supertasker may simply be down to your genetic "dice" rolling a double six, rather than snake eyes!

Will Listening to Music Improve My Concentration?

Listening to music nudges your brain during tedious work, but it's a myth that classical music makes you smarter.

First coined in 1991, the "Mozart Effect" became a craze among parents and students after a series of short experiments showed that some students performed slightly better in certain types of tests when taken shortly after a music lesson or listening to classical music. Newspapers loved the story, whipping up these findings into "listening to Mozart makes you smarter"—which was a bold stretch of the imagination.

Since then, further research has shown that while background music does give a slight boost to spatial reasoning (the ability to imagine and answer questions about 2-D and 3-D objects), it doesn't improve your score in IQ or academic tests. Even then, the improvement doesn't last long, and the music doesn't even need to be classical—any pleasant background sound helps you stay focused, and lively pop and rock tunes tend to come out best of all. So if you are undertaking spatial reasoning tasks such as repairing a gadget, reading a map, or video gaming, put on your favorite upbeat track.

How Often Should I Take a Break?

Dawn-to-dusk workaholics are not as productive as they boast. Like a muscle, the thinking brain needs recovery time, and it's important to appreciate its limits.

Whatever you are doing, your brain is whirring in one of three gears; each one has a unique firing pattern that puts different demands on its circuitry.

When something catches our attention, the watching system known as the "salience" network kicks in, firing in short pulses and readying us to take action. This intense state of alertness can be maintained for only a short time before reaction times nosedive.

When we concentrate, the "central executive" network takes over—the brain's bulky frontal regions crackling like lightning as we analyze and solve problems. Continuous concentration can be maintained for a maximum of about 80 minutes before brain networks start to get sluggish.

When we disengage fully from work, the mind freewheels to a wandering state, controlled by a group of brain cells called the "default mode" network. Only in this relaxed state can the brain's other systems start to rebuild their reserves.

If you can't take a proper break, do a task that calls for a different kind of thinking—although not as beneficial as switching off entirely, this will buy you a little more time before your weary brain cells give up the ghost.

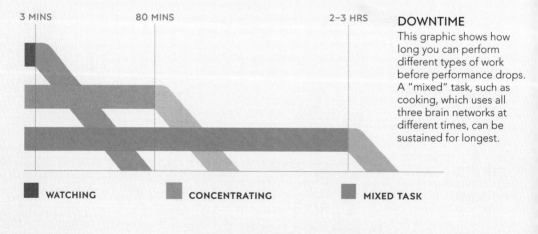

3 MINS   80 MINS   2–3 HRS

DOWNTIME

This graphic shows how long you can perform different types of work before performance drops. A "mixed" task, such as cooking, which uses all three brain networks at different times, can be sustained for longest.

■ WATCHING   ■ CONCENTRATING   ■ MIXED TASK

Why Am I So Easily Distracted?

It's in our nature to be easily distracted; any sudden movement or sound triggers an automatic reflex to look at it. This is a survival reflex called the "orienting response."

Our ancestors needed the "orienting response" reflex to instantly turn their attention to potential predators in the undergrowth. It's still useful to avoid everyday dangers such as reckless drivers—but not so much when working on constantly changing screens. There's no turning this life-saving reflex off, so that's why you need to mute pop-up notifications.

Some of our workspaces don't do us any favors, either—open-plan workspaces are full of visual and sound distractions that constantly activate your brain's "watching" (salience) network, causing your "concentrating" (executive control) network to stop and start. Seclude yourself in a side office or private cubicle to minimize distractions.

However, sometimes distractions are useful. Monotonous, repetitive work, such as production line work or data entry, can lull the brain into its inward-looking "wandering" state (default mode network). A little stimulation, such as music or drawing a doodle at your desk, is often enough to reactivate the other networks and prevent the mind from wandering too far so we don't miss something important.

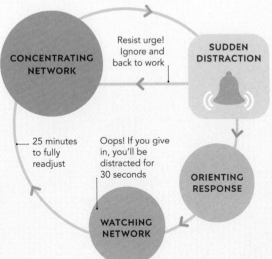

DON'T CHECK THAT NOTIFICATION!
When you are fully concentrating, if you allow a sudden distraction to switch on the other brain networks, it can take up to 25 minutes for you to regain your concentration.

CONCENTRATING NETWORK

Resist urge! Ignore and back to work

SUDDEN DISTRACTION

25 minutes to fully readjust

Oops! If you give in, you'll be distracted for 30 seconds

ORIENTING RESPONSE

WATCHING NETWORK

Why Do I Get the Best Ideas When I'm Not Trying?

You're strolling in the park when suddenly the solution to a tricky problem comes to you. When your guard is down, your unfettered brain is free to form insights.

When you're not thinking about anything in particular, your brain is far from idle—a sprawling web of cells called the default mode network (see page 70) is shuttling impulses across the many different brain regions. No longer tethered to narrow thinking processes, you can ponder the past and the future, fully empathize with others, and build new connections and associations. Such light-bulb moments have been behind many of humankind's greatest discoveries; for example, Albert

Einstein unraveled his theory of relativity after getting lost in his thoughts while doing routine work as a clerk.

Anxiety and stress are the enemy of aimless thought. Feeling under threat restrains the brain's "wandering" default mode network and instead nudges the brain toward its vigilant salience network. Writer's block is a mental trap brought on by becoming anxious about a lack of creativity. This becomes a vicious circle that makes it even more difficult to think creatively, upping the anxiety further.

If you're feeling blocked, take a break and relax so your brain switches back to its wandering network. Monotonous tasks, like doing dishes or driving, can calm the mind enough to bring on an epiphany, which is why cruising along the highway can ignite our best ideas.

Medial prefrontal cortex: thinking, analyzing, and making decisions

Posterior cingulate cortex: memories and emotions hub, planning for the future

ACTIVE AREAS OF BRAIN IN DEFAULT MODE NETWORK

THE DAYDREAMING BRAIN

When your mind drifts, your gray matter is sparking with activity and forming ideas. The prefrontal cortex lights up as you daydream, and the posterior cortex might be generating strong emotions.

How Can I Maximize My Creativity?

There are many ways you can encourage creativity, depending on the time of day, the space you work in, and how you take care of yourself.

Contrary to what you might expect, you are often at your creative best just when you think you are at your worst. This is because creativity and lateral thought flourish when your mind is in its wandering, default mode network, which is more likely when your concentrating, executive control network is running at low ebb. For night owls, creativity is maximal in the morning; for morning larks, the best ideas tend to come in the evening.

The three brain networks—wandering, watching, and concentrating—work together to develop your creativity. Learning new skills helps your brain form new pathways, encouraging these three networks to collaborate more effectively. Allow time for creativity and work in a space that encourages you to be creative, without trying to force it. Take regular breaks to prompt your brain to think outside the box. Get enough rest and sleep, since anxiety-inducing pressure will choke creativity.

CREATIVE THOUGHT PROCESS
Creative ideas and lateral thought follow a direction of travel through different brain networks, beginning with the crucial wandering network.

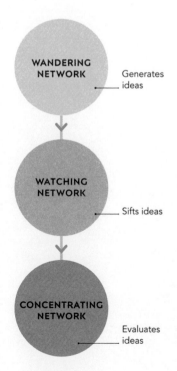

WANDERING NETWORK — Generates ideas

WATCHING NETWORK — Sifts ideas

CONCENTRATING NETWORK — Evaluates ideas

Is My Workplace Making Me Sick?

An office might seem a safe haven compared to a coal mine or building site, but poor air quality can cause nasty, health-threatening symptoms. The answer? Get a plant or two.

Poorly ventilated offices are at risk of causing "sick building syndrome" in which people suffer symptoms that worsen during the working day, including rashes, headaches, sneezing, coughs, and fatigue. Chemicals known as volatile organic compounds, released into the air from furniture, carpets, machinery, and cleaning fluids, can build up to toxic levels. Adding to this noxious mix are dust, mold, and bacteria.

Australian researchers tested different plants' abilities to remove airborne chemicals in offices. They found that three or more large plants per person in an office can indeed improve air quality by removing half of all VOCs, as well as stripping out nearly all carbon monoxide from the air.

BEST PURIFYING PLANTS

- Kentia palm (*Howea forsteriana*)
- Devil's ivy (*Epipremnum aureum*)
- Peace lily (*Spathiphyllum*)
- Umbrella tree (*Schefflera*)

As well as absorbing toxic substances, the leaves suck up carbon dioxide

Used in cleaning agents, varnish, paint remover

TOLUENE — Found in paint thinner

XYLENE

BENZENE — Found in plastics, cleaning fluid, synthetic fibers

N-HEXANE — Found in textiles

CLEAR THE AIR
Plants and soil microbes absorb many potentially harmful compounds; some of them are listed on the pot shown here.

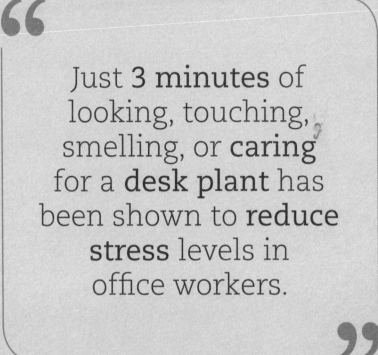

> Just **3 minutes** of looking, touching, smelling, or **caring** for a **desk plant** has been shown to **reduce stress** levels in office workers.

Why Can't I Get a Word in Edgewise in Meetings?

That punch-in-the-gut feeling of being cut off or ignored is something we've all experienced—and women suffer it more than men.

Research across cultures shows that men dominate conversations, interrupt more, and have their suggestions taken more seriously by others—even by women. Assertiveness by a woman in a male-dominated workplace is more likely to be viewed as "bossy" and "abrasive"; conversely, men who act identically are more likely to be termed "decisive" and "assertive."

Many self-help and business gurus have said that women's views are unfairly sidelined because their speech is too "feminine"—punctuated with phrases that are termed "softeners," such as "sort of," "just wanted to …", and "I'm sorry but…." They say these make the speaker sound hesitant and indecisive to others. Objective research shows, however, that this theory is mostly hot air. Men use this kind of speech just as much as women.

So why are men such verbal bulldozers in the workplace? Male dominance at work has less to do with language and biological authority, and

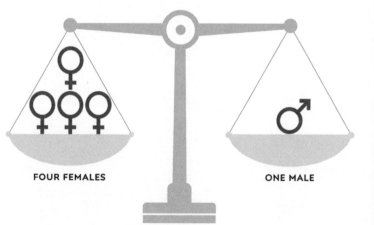

UNBALANCED
In a mixed-sex discussion group, women tend to get equal airtime only when the group has a ratio of at least four women for every man in the group.

FOUR FEMALES

ONE MALE

more to do with entrenched, global views of men having authority and taking command, while women are seen as more passive and family-focused. This work divide started around 10,000 years ago, when humans began farming in settlements, and whether we like it or not, these roles have seeped into the world's psyche: patients feel more assured when their surgeon is a man, and air passengers

WOMEN ARE **NOT CHATTIER** THAN **MEN**; BOTH **SPEAK** AROUND

16,000
WORDS PER DAY

say they are more relaxed when the pilot's voice they hear has a baritone rather than a soprano pitch.

Despite this, research shows that the most effective teams are mixed gender, and that strong female role models (especially in positions of leadership) help shatter stereotypes. We all have our part to play by being aware of this traditional norm and by striving to find and work with others who see the world differently to us.

PSYCHOLOGY OF THE GENDER DIVIDE

Unconscious prejudices are slow to uproot in societies. Humans are tribal; our unspoken social rules have been key in knitting together fragile communities over tens of thousands of years. Everyone conforms, and everyone is expected to conform. If we humans had not developed social norms, then we would have cooperated only haphazardly and not been able to form such stable societies.

Even though the world has been inching toward a more gender-balanced society, primal psychology still remains powerfully at play. Anyone who bucks the trend by acting differently to what has gone before risks a social backlash for defying the expectations of others.

We also suffer "confirmation bias" (see page 170), valuing those men and women who conform to stereotypes and dismissing those who don't as being unusual.

Even when our collective ideals shift, there is still a time lag before it affects how individuals actually live and work. Nevertheless, the choices we make today will have an impact on the accepted rules in our tribe. Each can be one small step in moving toward the world we want to live in tomorrow.

Are Male and Female Brains Wired Differently?

We all love to point out where we differ, but when it comes to our brains, research shows that there are far more similarities than differences.

We are told that men and women are so different, it's as if they came from separate planets. Martian men are stereotypically target-focused, assertive, and good at navigating; women from Venus are more empathetic, caring, and expert multitaskers. We are all fascinated by what makes the other sex tick, but back on Earth, when it comes to brains, much of what's been written about the sex divide is more science fiction than science fact.

Websites and news outlets have seeped scientific-sounding theories into common wisdom, such as the idea that women listen with both sides of their brain, whereas men use only one side; or that men and women navigate using "entirely different" brain regions. Some even claim that there is a "male brain" and a "female brain."

These ideas often have their roots in scientific research, but much of it is based on early experiments that picked out differences in our brains that were found later to be insignificant, or their results were misinterpreted or misreported. Scientists are suckers for

SPOT THE DIFFERENCE

These graphs are two of many that show the perceived chasm separating male and female brains is not so huge after all. When scientists compared regions of the brains in the sexes, scans showed that most brain regions are a similar size.

KEY

●—●—● Females

●—●—● Males

Most people have similar-sized amygdalas—the same pattern holds true for most brain regions

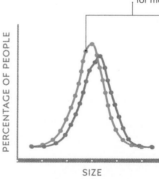

PERCENTAGE OF PEOPLE

SIZE

LEFT AMYGDALA

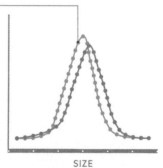

SIZE

RIGHT AMYGDALA

wanting to tell a story that will be the talk of the town—and the media are willing accomplices. Less headline-grabbing experiments that show little or no difference can get stuffed in the drawer, never to see the light of day.

So what does the science really say? From the eighth week in the womb, little boys' and girls' brains do start to develop slightly differently. Throughout our lives, the sex hormones testosterone, estrogen, and progesterone mold our individual physical and emotional development. Hormone level differences tweak the dial on characteristics such as aggression, pain threshold, stress response, and parent-child bonding, but each person is so unique that there is often more variation within each sex than there is between them.

Male and female brains don't differ significantly in size, either. Men's brains are slightly larger as a consequence of their larger bodies, and thanks to detailed scanning, we know that some brain parts differ in proportion between the sexes (see diagram, left), but the differences are too small to claim that there is such a thing as a "male brain" or a "female brain."

Most areas of mental functioning, behavior, and personality are the same in both sexes. What differences there are, such as in aggression levels, are usually driven by the differences in sex hormones such as testosterone after puberty.

SO IS IT NATURE OR NURTURE?

Recent research points to the historic sex divide actually being down to society, not science. When the magnifying glass of science reveals the workings of the brain, the accepted male and female stereotypes mostly vanish.

Some scientists now think that what differences there are between male and female brains—such as, say, in map reading—are the result, not of biology, but of thousands of years of brain training. The good news, however, is that the brain is great at learning new things—you can adapt and learn many new skills within a lifetime.

So it is logical that, if given the opportunity, men and women can learn skills stereotypical of the other sex very easily. For example, children who are given LEGO bricks to play with are likely to mature and have brains that have larger spatial cortexes, regardless of whether they are male or female.

Why Do I Feel Hungry So Soon After Breakfast?

You may think hunger is your body's way of telling you it needs more fuel—but it's more often than not just driven by your stomach's never-ending desire to be filled.

In evolutionary history, our ancestors survived and weathered potential famines by eating food whenever it was available, and our biology still reflects our food-craving past.

From the moment the stomach starts to empty its contents into the intestines, the urge to eat again begins. When your stomach deflates, its slippery walls release the food-craving hormone ghrelin, which sticks like syrup to the tiny appetite-controlling region of the brain. This triggers the primal need to eat, and as more and more ghrelin sticks, your hunger levels will steadily rise. Long-term stress and lack of good sleep can also trigger ghrelin release, dialing up appetite.

There are ways you can keep greedy ghrelin from wrecking your good intentions. Quick-digesting breakfasts will leave the stomach promptly and cause ghrelin to be released quickly, so cravings end up plaguing your morning. Instead, try to eat foods full of unrefined carbohydrates and fiber to ensure digestion is slower (see pages 36–37).

BALLOONING STOMACH

After eating, the stomach deflates and releases copious amounts of ghrelin, the hunger hormone, which tells your brain that you're hungry. When your stomach expands after a meal, less ghrelin is released, dialing down your appetite.

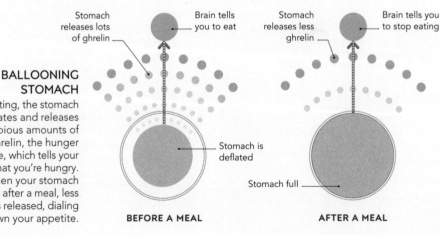

Stomach releases lots of ghrelin

Brain tells you to eat

Stomach is deflated

BEFORE A MEAL

Stomach releases less ghrelin

Brain tells you to stop eating

Stomach full

AFTER A MEAL

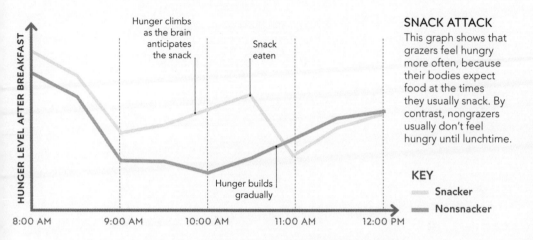

Hunger climbs as the brain anticipates the snack

Snack eaten

Hunger builds gradually

HUNGER LEVEL AFTER BREAKFAST

8:00 AM   9:00 AM   10:00 AM   11:00 AM   12:00 PM

SNACK ATTACK
This graph shows that grazers feel hungry more often, because their bodies expect food at the times they usually snack. By contrast, nongrazers usually don't feel hungry until lunchtime.

KEY

Snacker

Nonsnacker

Is Grazing the Healthiest Way to Eat?

Eating every three hours is seen by many as the best way to keep the brain ticking and the legs pumping. But is eating little and often really the key to good health?

Health advice often swings between pro- and anti-snacking, and currently snacking is the trend. For example, advertisements for cereal bars suggest they boost performance and that hungry means unhealthy, but it's a myth that we will "crash" if we don't eat every three or four hours (see page 96).

Some recent research suggests that continual grazing through the day is linked to an overly active immune system, although whether this is harmful to health isn't yet clear.

Snacking in itself neither helps weight loss nor causes weight gain. Allowing ourselves to get very hungry, however, when there are lots of high-calorie treats on hand is a temptation to our survival-seeking primal instincts. The signals that are released by the most ancient, animal-like parts of our brain in the hypothalamus when we are very hungry subvert our rational thinking so that we grab whatever is going to provide maximum fuel—such as the bag of chips and chocolate bar lurking in the desk drawer.

Do I Need to Drink Eight Glasses of Water a Day?

Carrying around a bottle of water is a badge of healthy living, and we're told to drink at least 8 glasses a day—however, this advice has more holes than a leaky bucket.

"Experts" urge us to drink water to flush out toxins and combat aging, but like so many health myths, the 8-glasses-a-day (or 2.5 liters) advice seems to have sprung from a misunderstanding. The US Food and Nutrition Board published advice in 1945 that a "suitable allowance of water for adults is 2.5 liters daily." Had thirsty health-seekers not gulped down this snippet right away, they would have read the next sentence, which stated that most of this will come from food. Healthy adults, they advised correctly, had no need to drink beyond their thirst. Nevertheless, the idea stuck, and the bottled water industry pours great efforts into continuing to persuade us to drink 2.5 liters a day.

On a day-to-day basis, forcing yourself to drink that much water is unnecessary and doesn't give credit for the body's highly attuned ability to keep you on an even keel. Your brain's thirst center continuously samples the blood to make you feel thirsty before you become dehydrated. Although overdrinking is rarely dangerous in normal circumstances, drinking large amounts of water during endurance sports may dilute body salts to perilously low levels, and can even be fatal.

Studies show there's no health benefit to drinking more than the amount we need to satisfy our thirst (except perhaps the extra exercise from more trips to the toilet!).

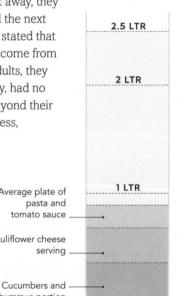

2.5 LTR

2 LTR

1 LTR

Average plate of pasta and tomato sauce

Cauliflower cheese serving

Cucumbers and hummus portion

HIDDEN SOURCES
You can easily receive a good proportion of your daily requirement of water from the food you eat.

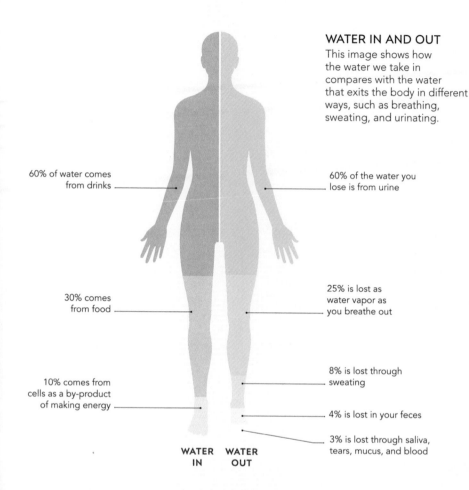

WATER IN AND OUT

This image shows how the water we take in compares with the water that exits the body in different ways, such as breathing, sweating, and urinating.

60% of water comes from drinks

60% of the water you lose is from urine

30% comes from food

25% is lost as water vapor as you breathe out

8% is lost through sweating

10% comes from cells as a by-product of making energy

4% is lost in your feces

3% is lost through saliva, tears, mucus, and blood

WATER IN   **WATER OUT**

Doctors recommend that adults living in a temperate climate and leading a sedentary lifestyle should drink about 6 cups (1.5 liters) of water-based drinks to make up for water lost through sweating, urination, and even the water vapor in their breath—the rest of the water you need will be obtained by eating a balanced diet.

You need to up your water intake if you're sweating from exercise, hot weather, or if unwell with a fever, diarrhea, or vomiting. The elderly may need encouragement to drink, because the thirst centers in their brains become sluggish in old age; similarly, young children are less aware of their thirst drive and need to have scheduled drink breaks through the day.

Should I Drink until My Pee Is Clear?

You may be familiar with the idea that the color of your pee can tell you whether you are drinking enough. But don't make the mistake of thinking that clearer is always better.

We may not know its name, but many of us are familiar with Armstrong charts from gym locker rooms or doctors' offices. Named after their scientist creator, they are designed to tell you whether you are dehydrated by comparing the color of your urine with yellowy-brown colored stripes.

The chart suggests that you should drink more if your urine matches the darker stripes and stop when your pee matches the palest colors. The chart is very useful as an early warning of dehydration, especially in the elderly, infirm, or very young. But it's a big mistake to think that paler is always better and that you should drink until urine runs completely clear. By doing this, there's a very good chance that you're putting yourself well on your way to fluid overload. If your urine is completely clear, it's an ominous sign that your kidneys are having to work overtime to remove excess water from your system.

COLOR MATCHING

It's healthiest for your pee to match the colors of the second or third colors on an Armstrong chart.

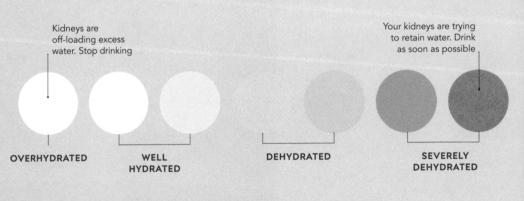

Kidneys are off-loading excess water. Stop drinking

Your kidneys are trying to retain water. Drink as soon as possible

OVERHYDRATED   WELL HYDRATED   DEHYDRATED   SEVERELY DEHYDRATED

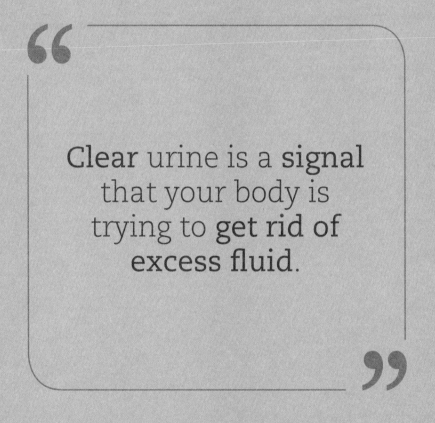

" Clear urine is a signal
that your body is
trying to get rid of
excess fluid. "

AFTERNOON

As the sun passes overhead, so the whirring
chemical cogs of our inner timepiece start to apply
the brakes. In the savanna, big cats lounge and fall
into their dozy siesta. We are not above nature's
rhythm: as we glide into lunchtime for a refuel, our
body and brain undergo a brief lull in activity.
Afterward, we are replenished to start the
next leg of our journey through the day.

What Makes a Good Lunch?

Lunch is a good opportunity to up your plant-based food intake and get your fill of important nutrients. A varied lunch is good for the body and boosts mood, too.

The only steadfast rule on what to have for lunch is to make sure you include a mixture of nutrient groups in your meal. Your decision-making abilities are better before lunchtime than soon after waking, giving you more mental ability to weigh up a healthy meal choice. However, when you're really hungry, the appetite control center in your brain's hypothalamus can scupper your good intentions; a spider's web

77% OF WORKERS HAVE THE SAME LUNCH EVERY DAY, SURVEYS REVEAL

of survival-based nerve pathways reaches into every corner of your being, putting your reward system on edge and firing up your "fight-or-flight" response.

Don't buy your lunch on an empty stomach; when ravenous, you will seek out high-energy foods that can be eaten with the least effort. With this neurological lack of self-control, you shouldn't be surprised if cakes, cookies, and chocolate turn up in the shopping basket. You can avoid this risk by pre-preparing a packed lunch.

Lunch offers more pleasure than breakfast. Your sense of taste has been improving throughout the morning, making middle-of-the-day fodder more flavorful. This is also why you're less likely to be happy if you eat exactly the same food every day—you're wasting your supercharged taste buds, and

NUTRIENT **GROUPS**

Each of the four main nutrient groups plays its own part in keeping you going.

- **Fiber** is important for a healthy gut and may even help reduce cholesterol.
- **Carbohydrates** provide your body's main source of energy.
- **Protein** is slow to digest so keeps you feeling fuller for longer. Your body uses the amino acids in protein to repair itself.
- **Unsaturated fats** are beneficial in small amounts—like coals on a fire, they give long-term energy and help the "gut brain" to decrease hunger.

since food and your "gut brain" are linked strongly with mood, making lunches more varied can even make you happier.

Nutrition science is always evolving, but you won't go far wrong if your lunches are full of natural, minimally processed foods. Nutritionally speaking, the less a food has been refined, manipulated, preserved, and flavor-enhanced, the better—subjecting food to an industrial process often removes or destroys fiber and nutrients and causes the food to be digested faster, making it less sustaining.

Olive and rapeseed oils contain healthy unsaturated fats

OILS

NUTS AND BEANS

Many beans, pulses, nuts, and soy-based foods such as tofu contain protein

Wholegrain brown bread, pasta, rice, noodles, oats, and cereals contain unrefined carbohydrates

WHOLE GRAINS

FRUITS AND VEGETABLES

PLANT-BASED LUNCH PYRAMID

Many kinds of plant sources such as root vegetables and fruit contain plenty of carbohydrates, fiber, vitamins, and minerals

GETTING THE RIGHT BALANCE

The digestive system is healthiest when it is fed a varied mix of food groups. The pyramid shows what proportions of each group to include in your meal. Making your lunch plant-based is a good way to reduce meat in your overall diet.

Is It Okay to Work While Having Lunch?

When the to-do list is endless, you might start to think you can't afford to take time out, but having lunch while working isn't sustainable in the long run.

Sadly, around half of office workers don't take time out for a lunch break. Not only are you adding to your total "sitting time" (see pages 100–101), but it's a false economy because your afternoon's productivity will be negatively affected. A hastily gobbled sandwich while checking your emails doesn't count, because far more important than refilling your abdominal food pouch is stepping away from where you spent your working morning. In the long term, if you have a habit of working through lunch, then you're more likely to be emotionally exhausted and suffer sleep problems, and you'll take more time off due to illness.

Leave your work behind at lunchtime to release the brain into its most relaxed firing patterns: memories form, emotions settle, thoughts consolidate, tense muscles relax, and stress responses calm. Wherever possible, taking a lunch break outdoors and around green spaces enhances its restorative effects. Bosses take note: a team lunch results in improved teamwork, morale, and productivity.

FALSE ECONOMY
It might feel like you're getting more done by taking lunch at your work station, but it's a short-term benefit. Studies show that working through lunch negatively affects productivity compared to taking a break away.

KEY
▬ Took lunch break
▬ Worked through lunch

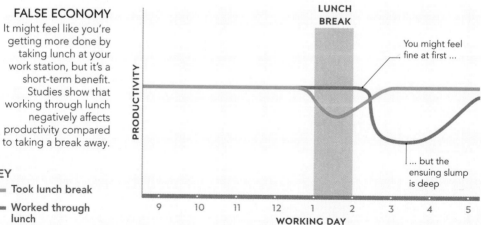

Is It Really Better to Eat Slowly?

Your mother was right. There's a time lag between when you finish a meal and when you feel full, and if you go back for more during this window, you may end up eating too much.

There are two signs that you are "full." The immediate feeling comes from your stomach—you'll start to feel bloated. As it fills, nerve receptors send out "full" signals to the brain. This is short-lived, though, since the stomach starts to deflate after about 5 minutes, and the "full" signals relent.

Liquids rush almost immediately through to the intestines. It's only when the second sign of fullness comes, as proteins, fats, and carbohydrates (including sugar) start to trickle into the small intestine, that we begin to feel properly fed. Incredibly, there are taste receptors in your intestines—just like those on the tongue!—and the gut brain starts to send out messages to the upstairs brain to dial down appetite when it gets this second taste.

Because of the delay between eating and the food being tasted by the gut, gobbling food quickly makes it easy to overeat. It's wise to wait a while to let your food settle before going for second helpings.

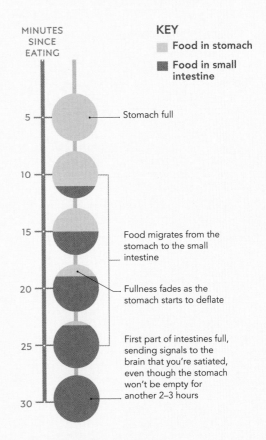

MINUTES SINCE EATING

KEY
- Food in stomach
- Food in small intestine

5 — Stomach full

10

15 — Food migrates from the stomach to the small intestine

20 — Fullness fades as the stomach starts to deflate

25 — First part of intestines full, sending signals to the brain that you're satiated, even though the stomach won't be empty for another 2–3 hours

30

DELAYED REACTION

This timeline shows the filling of the intestine after a meal. After you've finished, try not to eat more over the next 20–30 minutes.

I Want to Eat Healthily, So Why Do I Eat Junk Food?

The lure of the fast-food joint often proves too much—don't be too hard on yourself, though, because junk food contains an unholy trinity of the nutrients your body craves the most.

Your body is biologically hardwired to crave sugar, fat, and salt to survive potential famine. Sugar is released by the body as fast-acting energy; fat gives an incredibly concentrated supply of long-lasting fuel; and salt is essential for body-fluid balance. These were typically quite difficult foods for our hunter-gatherer ancestors to find, and no single naturally occurring food

A SUPERSIZED FAST-FOOD BURGER CAN **EXCEED** YOUR **DAILY FAT ALLOWANCE** BY

22%

contains these three enticements together. So when you get your hands on a fast-food burger, with its sweetened bun, sugary dressing, and meat loaded with salt and fat, a strong, triple-whammy biological craving rises up in you.

Compounding this, eating sweet-fatty-salty foods delivers a short but powerful dose of the rewarding brain hormone dopamine—the very same substance that makes you feel good after sex, winning the lottery, or watching your favorite sports team win a match. Dopamine is one of the main brain chemicals that drives addictions, so it's no wonder a habit of eating junk food can be difficult to drop.

WANT TO TRIUMPH OVER JUNK FOOD?

1

MAKE SURE YOUR DIET includes plenty of high-fiber vegetables to keep you sustained for longer and keep the hunger homone ghrelin at bay.

2

AVOID EATING WHEN STRESSED because the hunger hormone ghrelin surges powerfully as part of the body's stress response, which is why we are greedy for feel-good food after an intense day.

3

CHOOSE A LESS TEMPTING ROUTE HOME, because just traveling past a fast-food outlet sign can be enough to trigger your brain to release anticipatory pleasure hormones, long before you smell fried food!

And to make matters worse, the hormone responsible for hunger, ghrelin, also sticks itself to dopamine cells in the brain, making the prospect of eating that glistening, sugar-topped doughnut increasingly irresistible the hungrier we get. We long for it like a dog does a juicy bone. Our brains begin to anticipate the hormonal rewards so that even before the clock says it's snack time, the feel-good flight is already accelerating down the runway, and putting a stop on it gets harder and harder!

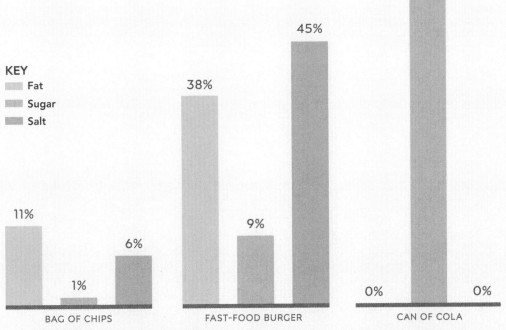

KEY

Fat

Sugar

Salt

78%

45%

38%

11%

9%

6%

1%

0%   0%

BAG OF CHIPS   FAST-FOOD BURGER   CAN OF COLA

PROPORTION OF DAILY RECOMMENDED AMOUNT OF FAT, SUGAR, AND SALT FOR ADULTS

EATING INTO YOUR ALLOWANCE

Fast food is quickly eaten and not filling but can swallow up a surprising proportion of your daily nutrition needs. A small bag of chips claims more than 10% of the recommended fat amount for adults, a burger almost half of the salt, and a can of cola more than three-quarters of your sugar total.

Why Is Sugar So Irresistible?

It's not your fault that you can't say no to sweet treats—you are fighting millions of years of evolution, which has conditioned you to crave sugar's instant rewards.

Sugar—no one needs it, but everyone loves it. Your body regards sugar as a true wonder food—you have taste buds devoted to sensing it and reward centers in the brain that generate intense pleasure when you eat it. Why? Because it does away with the hard graft of digestion. An apple delivers the same energy as a large spoonful of sugar but is disintegrated by the digestive system slowly, yielding a steady trickle of glucose over a few hours. Pure sugar, however, inundates the bloodstream within minutes. For 99 percent of our history, refined sugar didn't exist—unless our ancestors stumbled on a beehive, sugars were not part of their diet. In modern times, consumption has skyrocketed—and our bodies aren't cut out for a

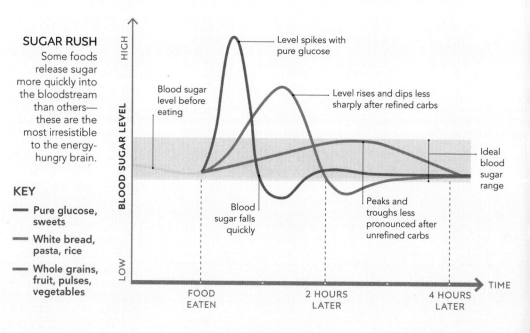

SUGAR RUSH
Some foods release sugar more quickly into the bloodstream than others—these are the most irresistible to the energy-hungry brain.

KEY

━━ Pure glucose, sweets

━━ White bread, pasta, rice

━━ Whole grains, fruit, pulses, vegetables

HIGH

BLOOD SUGAR LEVEL

LOW

Level spikes with pure glucose

Blood sugar level before eating

Level rises and dips less sharply after refined carbs

Ideal blood sugar range

Blood sugar falls quickly

Peaks and troughs less pronounced after unrefined carbs

TIME

FOOD EATEN

2 HOURS LATER

4 HOURS LATER

sustained sugar onslaught. With many of us living sedentary lives, sugar makes it easy to eat more food than we need, resulting in a bulging waistline. But more than making us fat, too much sugar has been implicated in many serious health conditions, including diabetes, heart disease, Alzheimer's, and some cancers.

So given that we're programmed to love sugars, are some healthier than others? Moderate intake of naturally

CONSUMPTION
OF SUGAR IN THE US HAS RISEN
2,255% SINCE 1700

occurring sugars, such as lactose in milk or fructose in fresh fruit, is fine. It's lots of added, refined sugars, such as sucrose (table sugar) and high-fructose corn syrup (HFCS), that really cause problems. Directly converted into fat within the liver, HFCS leads to fatty liver, furred arteries, and a high risk of diabetes, when the body can no longer keep high blood sugar in check.

If you really can't ignore those candy cravings, try indulging right after dinner. Sugars have an instant, if short-lived, appetite-curbing effect, so a little of something sweet can block the urge to continue eating, allowing time for the gut and brain to register that you are full.

BIG SUGAR SHIFTS THE BLAME

It was back in 1972, when British researcher John Yudkin published his book *Pure, White and Deadly*, that the warning was first sounded to the world about the health risks of eating too much sugar.

Cast out as a crackpot by the scientific world at large, Yudkin turned out to be on the money, yet his voice was comprehensively smothered by the power of the sugar industry.

Enticed by the big dollars of big sugar, health researchers were persuaded to redirect their efforts away from sugar toward uncovering the "evils" of a high-fat diet. Chief flag-waver for the fat-is-bad brigade was the (now much-critiqued) American researcher Ancel Keys, who poured scorn on dissenting scientists' findings.

Convinced by the weight of the evidence that (correctly) showed how diets high in *saturated* fats caused arteries to fur up and led to heart disease, government bodies worldwide shifted their guidelines. Before long, fats in general were branded as public health enemy number one. Sugar was sidelined as a lesser evil, while the nails were hammered instead into the coffin of the deep-fat fryer.

How Can I Avoid a Sugar Crash?

Many people fear that three hours without food risks running the gauntlet of suffering low blood sugar. But for most adults, the "sugar crash" is a fairy tale.

The "sugar crash" is a modern idea: in the mid-20th century, three meals a day was considered ideal, but in modern times, the idea has taken hold that we need to top up regularly to avoid slumps in energy. This snack culture is promoted, too, by corporate-sponsored research that suggests eating (and buying) snacks will boost performance.

You don't have to worry about crashing or your energy plummeting—unless you're diabetic or exercising hard for an hour or more, blood sugar rarely falls to levels that you can feel because your body takes care of it for you. The pancreas produces two useful hormones—glucagon and insulin—that dial down or push up sugar levels according to your body's needs. When they're creeping up, insulin pushes excess sugar into energy stores, first filling up short-term caches in our muscles and liver, then stowing the rest as fat. When sugar is low, glucagon drags sugar back out of these stores to keep your energy lines well supplied. Your body is amazingly good at regulating sugar and keeping energy levels balanced.

THE SUGAR POLICE

In most people, insulin and glucagon act as buffers for your blood sugar level, reacting to your food intake and energy output to keep levels within optimum limits.

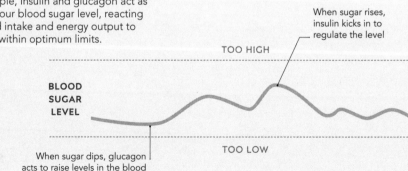

When sugar rises, insulin kicks in to regulate the level

TOO HIGH

BLOOD SUGAR LEVEL

TOO LOW

When sugar dips, glucagon acts to raise levels in the blood

SECRET SUGAR
It can be a shock to see how much hidden sugar there can be in processed foods. Just one serving of this fruit yogurt can push the limit of your daily sugar allowance.

How Much Sugar Can I Have, Then?

The WHO recommends five teaspoons of sugar a day. It's easy to keep track of the sugar we add to our tea, but it's important to watch out for less obvious sources.

Sugar itself is not the demon—the devil is in the dose. The WHO recommendation refers to refined sugars—not the sugars naturally contained in whole fruit and dairy products.

Obvious sources of added sugar are sweets and cakes, but it's worth checking how much sugar is in processed foods such as ketchup, spreads, bread, and ready meals, because you'll almost certainly find they contain more sugar than you thought—making it all too easy to accidentally go over the recommended daily limit. In fact, more than two-thirds of supermarket packaged goods have

some added sugar. Sugar can come in many guises—if you see dextrin or ethyl maltol on the list of ingredients, they're simply chemical names for types of sugar.

It's unfair to liken sugar to a drug such as cocaine, as many people and even some scientists now suggest. Sweetness is a basic taste that gives us happiness and satisfaction via a hearty squirt of dopamine in the brain's reward areas.

You can live without refined sugar, but there isn't any evidence that ridding every trace of it from your diet will make you healthier—so just enjoy it in moderation.

Can I Train Myself Not to Have a Sweet Tooth?

Your sweet tooth is written in the stars: your genes determine whether you find sweet foods especially irresistible. But that doesn't mean you must be at the mercy of your sweet tooth.

In most people, the liver produces a hormone called FGF21 (fibroblast growth factor 21) that applies the brakes to sugar cravings. However, some people are genetically hardwired to produce less of this hormone. If that's you, you're more likely to have a sweet tooth—and also get greater pleasure from alcohol!

You have thousands of taste receptors peppered all over your tongue, and their sensitivity to certain tastes (including sweetness) is unique to you like a fingerprint. Whether you

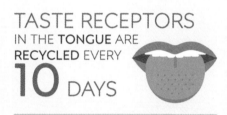

TASTE RECEPTORS IN THE **TONGUE** ARE **RECYCLED** EVERY **10** DAYS

find sweet foods very sickly or coriander soapy is down to the roll of the genetic dice. You may find you gradually lose your sweet tooth—taste receptors are recycled every 10 days. As we get older, these regenerated taste buds become progressively dulled.

The pleasure you get from any particular food is also knitted to your emotional memory of when you last ate it—and that's something you have agency over. If you enjoyed a decadent chocolate dessert during a special moment with a loved one, that may well be enough to turn an occasional cake eater into a cookie monster. Try nonsweet snacks to pair enjoyable memories with new foods.

WANT TO KEEP YOUR **SWEET TOOTH IN CHECK?**

1

CUT DOWN ON SUGAR—within a week or two, you get just as much pleasure from lower sugar alternatives.

2

FIND A FAVORITE SAVORY SNACK, eat it, and savor the feeling to tie it in to your emotional register, making it more likely you'll want to eat it again.

"

Those of us who have **fewer sweet-sensitive** tongue **receptors** need **more sweetness** in order to **appreciate** the taste.

"

Is Sitting Down "the New Smoking"?

Studies show that a sedentary lifestyle can slash life expectancy by seven years, but exactly what harm are you doing by lounging on the sofa after work?

The shocking claim that sitting down is as unhealthy as smoking, touted by journalists and scientists alike, makes you sit up and think twice about your daily routines, but you should blow smoke on the comparison. It is true that, just as smokers can't repair all long-term lung damage by giving up, you won't be able to undo all the ill effects of prolonged sitting just by doing some exercise. However, smoking is in an unhealthy league of its own. Few smokers are lucky enough to get into old age without suffering some kind of lung disease or cancer, whereas many desk workers lead a perfectly healthy life. Smoking increases your risk of dying each year by an average of 180 percent, while sitting down all day leads to a 25 percent increase.

Most people in developed countries now spend most of their waking hours on their posterior, and it's taking a toll on our physical health. Even someone who exercises for 45 minutes each day probably spends most of their remaining

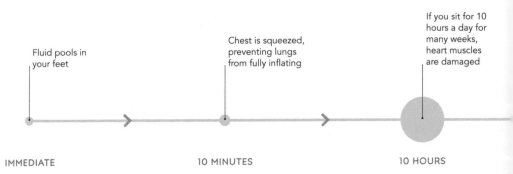

Fluid pools in your feet

Chest is squeezed, preventing lungs from fully inflating

If you sit for 10 hours a day for many weeks, heart muscles are damaged

IMMEDIATE   10 MINUTES   10 HOURS

DANGERS OF SITTING

Your body is built to move: its 200-plus bones, connected by 360 joints, clothed in a jacket of 700 muscles, hold you upright and propel you forward. This timeline shows how prolonged sitting compromises the body in different ways.

16 hours sitting. Commuting, working, and eating are all done in a seat, and evenings are often spent unwinding in front of a screen.

The more hours you sit every day, the more harm you do to your body.

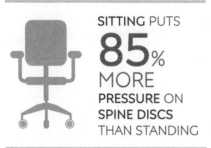

SITTING PUTS

85%
MORE
PRESSURE ON
SPINE DISCS
THAN STANDING

All this sluggishness cramps our concentration, increases fatigue, puts strain on the heart and circulation, alters the body's internal chemistry, and accelerates fatty buildup in arteries.

WANT TO **LIMIT THE TIME** SPENT **ON YOUR BEHIND?**

1

TRY A STANDING DESK to improve blood flow, facilitate creative thinking, and boost alertness. If you can't do that, take every opportunity to stand up—for instance, to speak to a colleague, make a call, or get a drink.

2

GO FOR A FIVE-MINUTE WALK every hour, which will cancel out many of sitting's negative health effects.

3

FIND MORE ACTIVE WAYS TO UNWIND such as yoga, cooking, or DIY to balance leisure time spent on the couch and encourage your brain to release mood-boosting hormones.

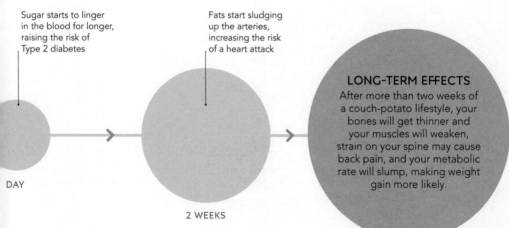

Sugar starts to linger in the blood for longer, raising the risk of Type 2 diabetes

Fats start sludging up the arteries, increasing the risk of a heart attack

LONG-TERM EFFECTS
After more than two weeks of a couch-potato lifestyle, your bones will get thinner and your muscles will weaken, strain on your spine may cause back pain, and your metabolic rate will slump, making weight gain more likely.

DAY

2 WEEKS

How Can I Avoid the Post-Lunch Slump?

After a large meal, your digestive system is calling the shots, turning you into a sleepy shadow of your morning self. But there are ways you can bargain with biology.

Hunger makes the mind alert—this is a survival necessity handed down from our ancestors, who needed to keep going while searching for food. Today, this lends us a little concentration boost leading up to lunch.

After a meal, the arteries widen so that there is a healthy blood supply for the gut to squeeze and extract the nutrients. Becoming a food-processing machine is hard work—and this surge of blood goes hand in hand with the urge to put head to pillow. The

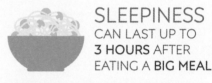

SLEEPINESS CAN LAST UP TO **3 HOURS** AFTER EATING A **BIG MEAL**

instigator of this so-called food coma (or postprandial somnolence, to give it its formal name) is the "gut brain." It releases sleep-inducing hormones, including cholecystokinin, so that you move less and your energy resources can instead go into the hard work of digestion.

After a big lunch, sleepiness can come on after about 20 minutes and last for hours, so if sharp thinking is called for in the early afternoon, a hearty midday meal is going to make that more challenging. Stay off the roads after lunch, or be cautious when driving, because there's a spike in automobile accidents at this time, thanks to all those drowsy drivers. Exercising after eating won't help you stay alert—the squashing and shaking of a food-bloated stomach will make you feel nauseous but no less sleepy.

WANT TO **AVOID FALLING ASLEEP** AT YOUR DESK?

1

KEEP YOUR LUNCH light so you aren't overwhelmed by sleepy gut hormones.

2

GET OUTDOORS—daylight (even on cloudy days) sends signals to your body clock to stay awake.

3

OR YOU COULD just go with nature. Studies show that even 5 minutes of shut-eye can be good for you.

The only way to lessen the slump is to eat less for lunch. The gut will release more sleep hormones when it is overfilled with food. Providing you eat enough during the day, you can minimize the disruptive effects of digestion and sleep hormones by keeping lunches light (see below).

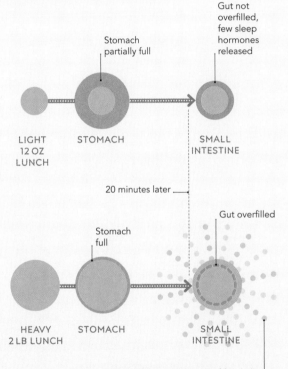

Gut not overfilled, few sleep hormones released

Stomach partially full

LIGHT
12 OZ
LUNCH

STOMACH

SMALL
INTESTINE

20 minutes later

Gut overfilled

Stomach full

HEAVY
2 LB LUNCH

STOMACH

SMALL
INTESTINE

Filled with a large amount of food, the gut releases sleep-inducing hormones

IT'S THE LITTLE THINGS

This shows the passage of a meal, first through the stomach and on to the gut (intestines). Sleep hormones are only released when the gut is very full—a lighter meal of around 12 oz (350 g) of both food and drink will help keep you alert in the afternoons.

THE NOT-SO SINFUL SIESTA

The 9–5 work ethic is completely at odds with the body clock; you are built for two sleeps each day, not one. Sleeping every six to eight hours is the norm in nature—chimpanzees and dolphins do it, and even insects have downtime in the hours after midday. Coinciding with the hottest hours when hard labor would risk overheating and dehydration, this rhythm is etched into your DNA, regardless of the climate you live in today.

Many cultures across the globe, including those in the Middle East, Asia, and South America, all have siesta culture in their history. It's western Europe and the US that live under the shadow of the "protestant work ethic." Starting in the 12th century, strict religious leaders preached that daytime sleep was an unnecessary, sinful luxury.

But by unpicking the afternoon nap routine that has been seamlessly woven into the tapestry of many traditional cultures, we in the West risk impairing our mental clarity and missing out on its health benefits (see pages 104–105).

How Long Is the Ideal Power Nap?

A daytime nap seems to be all the rage again. Your body clock would approve—it is built for two sleeps a day, and different nap lengths offer you different benefits.

In many parts of the world, napping or simply resting in the afternoon is a normal part of daily life (see page 103).

Even very short amounts of shut-eye in the daytime can have marked effects. Many experts recommend that it should be 15 minutes, with a cup of coffee just before to give a boost on waking, although there isn't a one-size-fits-all approach.

If putting your feet up in the middle of the day is impossible, at least use the time for the least mentally demanding, low-risk tasks: informal meetings, train commutes, cleaning, or a mundane job you've been putting off.

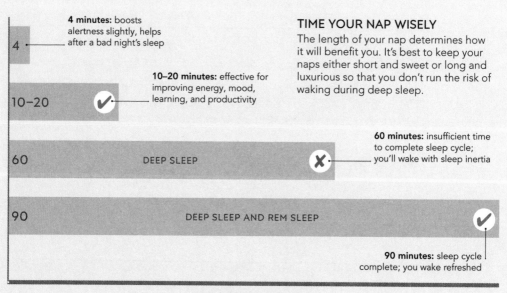

4 minutes: boosts alertness slightly, helps after a bad night's sleep

10–20 minutes: effective for improving energy, mood, learning, and productivity

60 minutes: insufficient time to complete sleep cycle; you'll wake with sleep inertia

90 minutes: sleep cycle complete; you wake refreshed

4

10–20

60 — DEEP SLEEP

90 — DEEP SLEEP AND REM SLEEP

SLEEP TIME IN MINUTES

TIME YOUR NAP WISELY
The length of your nap determines how it will benefit you. It's best to keep your naps either short and sweet or long and luxurious so that you don't run the risk of waking during deep sleep.

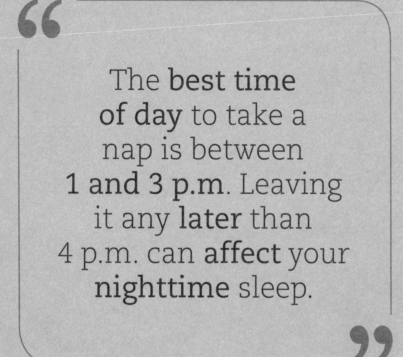

" The **best time of day** to take a nap is between **1 and 3 p.m**. Leaving it any **later** than 4 p.m. can **affect** your **nighttime** sleep. "

Should I Trust My Gut Instinct?

When facing a dilemma, we sometimes feel "drawn" a particular way. But whether or not we should heed our intuition comes down to hard science.

Trusting your gut feelings is often seen as a mark of the brave, successful, and gifted. These impulses don't arise from your gut, of course, but are prelearned responses driven by the emotion center, the amygdala, in your brain.

Emotional memories completely bypass your analytical frontal lobes, which is why they seem to "come out of nowhere." Your emotional amygdala constantly chatters with the hippocampus—the orchestrator of

memories—to provide you with the best guess on what's about to happen, based on your past experiences. This is why you should trust your gut instincts only in areas of your life that are familiar. For example, if you head up an estate agency, then your amygdala and hippocampus will feed you "gut instincts" based on your years of experience of the local market. However, your gut is likely to mislead if you enter a completely different

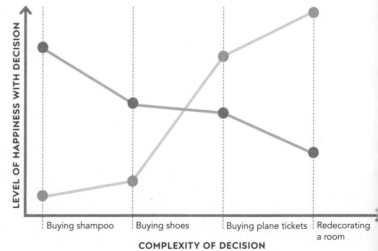

DECISIONS, DECISIONS
This graph illustrates that the more complex the decision, the more likely it is that your instinct will be successful. When a problem increases in scale and complexity, it's actually better to go with your gut because you risk overanalyzing the issue.

KEY
- Conscious deliberation
- Gut instinct

LEVEL OF HAPPINESS WITH DECISION

Buying shampoo · Buying shoes · Buying plane tickets · Redecorating a room

COMPLEXITY OF DECISION

industry, such as food retail—since your intuition is refined in an emotional furnace of trial and error, most of these emotional memories probably don't apply here. In unfamiliar territory, it's best to rely on the expertise of others more experienced than you—regardless of your age.

Your hunches can also be trusted only in areas of life that are fairly predictable and repeatable, such as flying, driving, games of chess, or video games. If there are too many variables, confidence in your gut is a recipe for failure: investors, for instance, are often misled by their intuition—stock markets do not follow patterns and are notoriously skittish and unpredictable.

In some instances, it might be worth sidelining your gut. Quiz show contestants often experience a psychological phenomenon called the "first instinct fallacy"—that you should trust your first hunch when presented with multiple choices. When faced with a set of options, you're better off weighing up the answers rather than picking the first one that appeals.

Professional intuition can be honed over time. An experienced chef knows when to take the frying pan off the heat while doing three other tasks at the same time because their emotional memories are fine-tuned to remember that stressful time when they *did* burn the onions. The gut instincts of novice chefs will be a bit wobbly at first—but they'll get there.

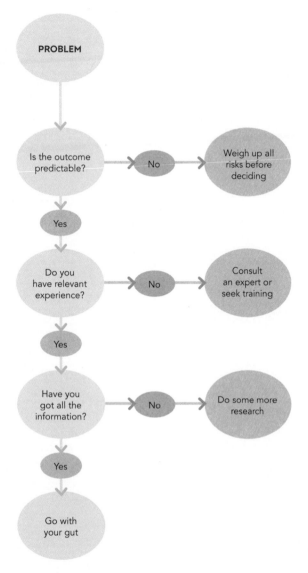

PROBLEM

Is the outcome predictable? → **No** → Weigh up all risks before deciding

Yes

Do you have relevant experience? → **No** → Consult an expert or seek training

Yes

Have you got all the information? → **No** → Do some more research

Yes

Go with your gut

WANT TO FOLLOW YOUR GUT?
Even the finest-tuned instinct can benefit from a bit of science. You can use the flow chart to help you decide whether going with your gut is a good idea by interrogating the factors surrounding each decision.

Are We All Really Getting More Stressed?

Modern life's pressures can feel like they are increasing, but science reveals that it's the nature of the stress we suffer today, rather than the amount, that has changed.

Before the 1940s, the only people who talked about "stress" were engineers describing whether the struts of a bridge would hold up. Today, "stress" is a vague catchall term for all of the many challenges you might face in life: you may have stress at home, be stressed out by work, and the anxiety you feel around hospitals or before exams can be "stressful." If you believe the headlines, the world is the most stressed out it's ever been—and we are fretting our way into an early grave.

Pick up any stress-management book or tap into a healthy-living website and you will encounter the classic stress story that we all undergo the "fight-or-flight" survival response and its accompanying deluge of hormones when stressed. However, the body is far more sophisticated than we give it credit for. No two "stresses" are the same: being punched in the gut triggers a different biological response to the turmoil of a feud with a neighbor or the worry over a delayed paycheck. Each demand (or "stressor") placed on you has its own survival response.

Different kinds of stress cause the body's defensive systems to react in different ways; for example, a brief stress response triggers helpful infection-fighting chemicals, whereas longer-term trauma can cause virus-attacking white blood cells to stop multiplying. Your responses also vary with age, past experiences, general health, and any medical conditions. You undergo the most drastic fight-or-flight responses only if you're threatened or physically injured.

"Stress" has become such a fuzzy term, it's no wonder we think there's more of it in the world. While it can be a useful way to understand our responses to mental and physical challenges, labeling every negative experience as "stress" risks impoverishing our experience of the richness of what it is to be human.

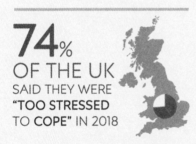

74%
OF THE UK
SAID THEY WERE
**"TOO STRESSED
TO COPE"** IN 2018

TYPE	POSSIBLE CAUSES	PATTERN OF STRESS RESPONSE
ACUTE TIME-LIMITED STRESSOR	The sudden pressure of public speaking or being put on the spot.	Pressure peaks and dips very quickly
BRIEF NATURALISTIC STRESSOR	A foreseen demand, such as taking an exam or meeting a work deadline.	Pressure builds slowly, then diminishes quickly
STRESSFUL EVENT	Bereavement or experiencing a major natural disaster.	Pressure recedes gradually after the event
CHRONIC STRESSOR	A draining job, messy divorce, or responsibility, such as caring for a loved one.	Pressure rises, falls slightly, then rises again
DISTANT STRESSOR	The recurring trauma of past events, such as being abused as a child or witnessing the death of a fellow soldier during war.	Original event · Trigger · Trigger · Pressure recurs when original event is recalled

THE MANY FACES OF STRESS

This chart sets out the different types of stress, characterized in terms of how they affect us and how long they last.

Is There a Quick Way to Calm My Nerves?

When you need to dial down your body's fight-or-flight response and still those trembling muscles, reassure your brain with some simple deep breathing.

The starter engine for your inner emergency alarm is an almond-shaped brain region called the amygdala, which screens what you see, hear, smell, feel, and think for potential threats to life and limb. The alarmed amygdala triggers a surge of adrenaline then a rush of blood sugar, readying the muscles for action. Your muscles may be so primed for action that they can start to shake—useful for our ancestors to make a quick getaway when hunted by predators, not so useful when you're trying to steer smoothly during a driving test!

It's possible to stop the shakes by training the brain pathways to realize that the threat is not dangerous. One of the simplest ways is to breathe deeply: inhale for four seconds, hold for four seconds, then exhale for four seconds. Unlike heart rate and blood pressure, which are out of your conscious control, breathing obeys your will. By forcing your lungs to expand and contract slowly, reassuring messages are relayed to the amygdala, calming you down.

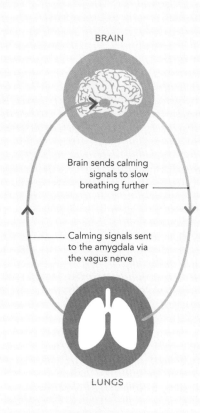

BRAIN

Brain sends calming signals to slow breathing further

Calming signals sent to the amygdala via the vagus nerve

LUNGS

CALMING CYCLE

When you consciously slow your breathing, you set up a cycle—the brain receives a message, it sends out calming signals and dials down stress hormones, and your breathing slows even more.

How Can I Manage Worrying Thoughts?

Even with the best laid plans, sometimes exams or impending deadlines can consume your mind. You can persuade your brain to feel less anxious, though.

Consistent, worrying thoughts about an impending event ramp up your amygdala's sensitivity, setting you up for a cycle of fretful ruminations that play out on repeat. When the amygdala is on high alert, the brain's greatest asset—the rational "executive" thinking networks—go silent, making us blind to the madness of our repeated irrational fears, leaving us to fret over impossible catastrophes or imagined arguments.

Also, perpetual wonderings about the past and what could have been—mistakes made, opportunities missed—slide your emotional limbic system toward a depressed state. Neurons that fire together, wire together: each time any thought—good or bad—is repeated, that crackling channel of electricity strengthens as they move and mold themselves around this route.

Over time, repeated thinking patterns become trodden out like a clear footpath through a field of wheat, at which point they become so familiar that they are second nature to us.

Breaking out of a mental tornado of emotional destruction, even when well entrenched, can be achieved by forcing the rational, executive networks to fire up. Combined with slow, deep breathing (see opposite page) and following a mind-calming bedtime routine for good sleep (see pages 226–227), plenty of practice can cut the fear off at its source. Science shows us a few tricks listed below with which you can do this.

WANT TO QUELL YOUR **INNER WORRYWART?**

1

REHEARSE CALM PATTERNS OF THINKING long before the amygdala anticipates a threat so that you carve out a familiar, peaceful pathway that is well away from anxiety alley.

2

DO SOMETHING—science shows that simple problem-solving can fire up the logical thinking networks.

3

FOCUS ON SOMETHING TANGIBLE outside yourself, such as counting the leaves on a plant, to help you fall into a calmer pattern of thinking.

How Can I Deal with Constant Stress?

You might be managing the drip-drip demands of constant deadlines, crying children, and rocky relationships for now, but beware—you're risking long-term damage.

Recurrent, relentless demands and uncertainties really can harm your health. The body's fight-or-flight response is a primal sledgehammer reaction that was a lifesaver for fending off predators but is now utterly out of proportion for cracking the small nuts of modern life's trials. With your emergency systems primed for a catastrophe, your body's internal chemistry is stretched to its limits. When fight-or-flight and stress hormones surge repeatedly over many days and weeks, it can cause damage to your internal organs, circulatory system, and brain (see opposite).

Coping strategies are often the go-to technique for dealing with repeated or long-term stress, and many of these are critical for quelling an overactive fight-or-flight response, offering you essential time to relax and reflect. They might include making to-do lists, exercise, yoga, meditation, breathing exercises, or even just "me time"—but they're all just an ice pack for soothing the fever and are rarely the cure. The best solution to never-ending pressures is to uproot the source and reframe how you think about the underlying problem.

If relentless pressure is putting your body on high alert, then you won't be able to see beyond the immediate crisis. By seeking advice from a trusted friend or family member, fresh perspectives and solutions often appear. There is also measurable evidence that working through problems with a professional counselor will let you unpick destructive thoughts and habits, as well as make practical steps to alleviate near-constant stress.

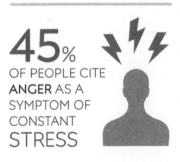

45%
OF PEOPLE CITE
ANGER AS A
SYMPTOM OF
CONSTANT
STRESS

BRAIN is stuck in its vigilant "watching" network leading to persistently low mood, anxiety, and destructive thought patterns

HEART RATE, blood pressure, and breathing are consistently elevated, risking health problems such as a heart attack or stroke

IMMUNE SYSTEM is tipped off-balance, causing bone marrow to pump out white blood cell types that fur up arteries and worsen allergies

BLOOD DIVERTED from digestive system toward muscles causes appetite loss and indigestion

WHEEL OF MISFORTUNE

Experiencing constant stress can feel like being caught in a never-ending loop of miserable symptoms, each feeding into the other. This constant state of high alert takes its toll all over the body.

CORTISOL no longer surges in the morning (see page 15), leaving you "burnt out"

CONSTANT FLOW of energizing hormone adrenaline slows digestion and causes symptoms of irritable bowel syndrome and other digestive problems

BODY CLOCK rhythms (see pages 22–23) become muted over time, leading to disrupted sleeping patterns

FUEL STORES have surplus energy, which gradually accumulates around internal organs as fat

Can Stress Ever Be Good for Me?

If you have ever felt the motivational push of stress, you'll know it can have its benefits. There's a fine balance to be kept between "good" and "bad" stress, however.

The natural "stress" hormones your body produces, and their effects on the body), are vital in providing you with the energy, strength, and single-mindedness to overcome physical and mental challenges. If your body can't produce enough cortisol to sustain you, then you'll be weak and fatigued. Without cortisol, your blood pressure and blood sugar will drop, you will be thirsty, and a sudden injury, infection, or bout of strenuous exercise could even lead to sudden death.

Not only is a stress response key to keeping you alive, but moderate pressure in daily life can do you good; regular pulses of adrenaline and cortisol when you're excited, motivated, or exercising improve concentration and provide small boosts in your mood.

However, constant and extreme demands will always be harmful (see pages 112–113), and if you're always falling ill when away from the stressor (see opposite), then that stress is doing you no good at all.

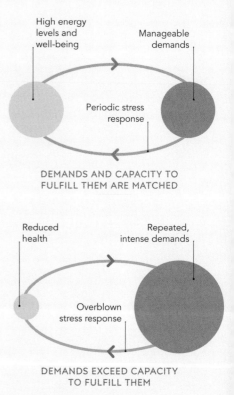

High energy levels and well-being

Manageable demands

Periodic stress response

DEMANDS AND CAPACITY TO FULFILL THEM ARE MATCHED

Reduced health

Repeated, intense demands

Overblown stress response

DEMANDS EXCEED CAPACITY TO FULFILL THEM

BALANCED DEMANDS

When life is manageable, the stress response is invigorating and sustaining. But when your demands seem to exceed your capacity, the stress response is ever-present and damaging.

Why Am I Always Ill When I Stop Working?

The freight train of coughs and aches you're hit with when you stop working is "leisure sickness." The plaster your body had put on invisible wounds has been ripped off.

When the phone won't stop pinging, a deadline is looming, and the children are screaming, invigorating stress hormones and the fight-or-flight buzz give the body's immune system a metaphorical shot in the arm. But take away the chemical stimulation, and suddenly the body is left open for an infection to strike.

Adrenaline and a hyped-up fight-or-flight state can also mask existing pain and ailments—not unlike the way that, if you fall and break your leg, you won't feel the pain until minutes or hours later. In the hecticness of life, it's possible that you have unknowingly been in the throes of fighting an infection or suffering an illness. Only when you take the foot off the pedal are the floodgates to muted aches and pains opened.

"Sickness behavior" is a well-evolved survival strategy: when the coast is clear and the body needs to fight an illness, you hunker down somewhere safe (away from sharp-toothed predators), do nothing (to use all your energy for fighting an infection and getting well), withdraw from everyone else (so you don't spread infection), and you feel more pain (so that you are attentive to your injuries).

Although few medical researchers have given leisure sickness the time of day, it seems that around 1 in 30 people suffer from it. Suffering every time you take a vacation may be your body's way of warning you that your lifestyle is beyond what can be sustained indefinitely. Plowing on may risk everything tumbling down in the form of a serious physical or mental health condition, which could include depression, burnout, or a long-term pain syndrome. Locate the stressor and consider a lifestyle change, such as a new job or new daily routine.

PERFECTIONISTS ARE 28% **MORE LIKELY** TO SUFFER **LEISURE SICKNESS**

How Much Time Should I Spend in the Sun?

Like plants, humans need sunlight to grow—but we need to balance this with protecting our skin from the sun's fearsome strength.

Like a stretchy covering of solar panels, the outermost layer of your skin harnesses the sun's ultraviolet (UV) rays to create the life-essential vitamin D.

Unfortunately, this type of UV ray called UVB has the same skin-burning frequency that causes skin cancer, wrinkles, and eye damage. Sunscreen offers some protection, but it also blunts vitamin D production. Like any medicine, some sunlight is good—but not too much, especially if you're fair-skinned. Our skin tone comes from melanin, a substance that acts like a biological bulletproof vest to shield our skin's precious DNA by absorbing slugs of UV light and dissipating its powerful punch as harmless warmth.

The darker your skin, the more UV-blocking melanin you have, so you need more sunlight than a fairer-skinned person to produce enough vitamin D. Darker-skinned people living in latitudes where the sun is weaker should consider taking vitamin D supplements, especially in winter.

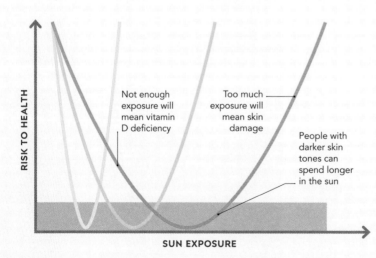

RISK TO HEALTH

Not enough exposure will mean vitamin D deficiency

Too much exposure will mean skin damage

People with darker skin tones can spend longer in the sun

SUN EXPOSURE

MELANIN SHIELD

There is a sweet spot of safe sun exposure—too little and you risk vitamin D deficiency; too much and you risk skin damage. Those with darker skin—and more melanin—can spend longer in the sun, but melanin can't protect you indefinitely.

KEY

▦▦▦ Fair skin tones

▦▦▦ Medium skin tones

▬▬▬ Dark skin tones

▦▦▦ Safety zone

Why Can't I Think Straight on a Hot Day?

Constantly active and churning out heat, the brain is already fighting to stay cool—so on a really warm day, it can easily crash and burn.

The brain is a demanding organ: its 90 billion electrically active brain cells are fussy about temperature, and they start to misfire and suffer damage if body temperature rises by just 3–4°F.

Your prefrontal cortex, or "thinking" region near the front of your brain, is particularly vulnerable—that's why heat stroke causes wooziness, muddled thinking, and confusion. On a hot day, your reaction times won't drop much and you'll be able to remember simple things such as a phone number, but anything more complicated than that—like paying close attention, driving, or solving a tricky problem—becomes progressively more difficult as your prefrontal cortex buckles in the heat.

Symptoms of heat exhaustion can involve dizziness, fainting, vomiting, and even seizures. Young children's brains are extra heat-sensitive.

If you live in warmer climes, then your body will usually be better adapted to get rid of excess heat. The body's go-to climate control methods are flushing the skin, where the blood rushes to the surface to release heat, and sweating, which cools you down by drawing heat from the body as the sweat evaporates.

It's not just our brains that dislike the heat; our muscles perform more poorly, too—it's better to leave hard, physical work for when the temperature is 68°F (20°C) or below.

FOR EVERY 1° ABOVE **77°F**, OUR MENTAL **ABILITY** WILL DROP BY ABOUT**2**%

HOW TO **KEEP YOUR HEAD ON A HOT DAY**

1

DRINK LOTS OF FLUIDS—you can lose up to 2 quarts (2 liters) of water per hour through sweating.

2

SLOW DOWN—exercising and physical labor put extra stress on the body and push body temperature up even higher.

3

SEEK SOME BREEZE—moving air, from a fan or an open window, will help sweat evaporate, accelerating its cooling effect.

Why Has My Teenager Turned into an Alien?

Your child may have suddenly become a moody mutant, but science lifts the lid on the dramatic brain transformations during this most misunderstood part of our lives.

Many parent-child misunderstandings arise because a teen's body and brain don't grow in harmony. Adolescence— the total period of mental transition from childhood to adulthood— takes longer than puberty, its physical equivalent. In fact, the brain is in adolescence from the age of 9 to the mid-20s. The law may say that they're adults at 18, but their heads are only half-cooked! The adolescent brain is a work in progress. It's not an overgrown child brain, nor is it an underdeveloped adult brain—MRI scans have revealed it is unique in its flexibility and capacity to learn.

Changing in shape, structure, and internal chemistry, your teenager's maturing brain is an easily excitable, socially sensitive machine that drinks in life experiences. In early childhood,

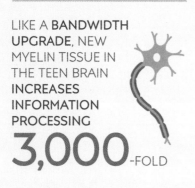

LIKE A **BANDWIDTH UPGRADE**, NEW MYELIN TISSUE IN THE TEEN BRAIN **INCREASES INFORMATION PROCESSING**

3,000-FOLD

gray matter on the brain's rippled surface (where the computing happens) inflated in size, sprouting millions of interconnected microscopic branches. However, by the ages of 12–14, that gray matter needs trimming back for efficient adult thought to bloom. Gray matter shrinks at first as unused brain pathways are cut, in much the same way that pruning a rose bush allows larger, stronger branches to develop. During this time of profound brain changes, your teenager can be prone to misjudgments and impulsive behavior.

Sex hormones often get the blame for a teen's erratic moods—but they're only part of the story. The brains of adolescents develop in a back-to-front order: the inner, emotional circuitry becomes adultlike long before the self-controlled, thinking regions in the brain's frontal lobes do. With the swirl of emotion-conveying tissue deep within the brain firing on all cylinders, teens' emotions have an adult intensity but without the measured restraint of a fully formed frontal lobe. A teen will suddenly know what they want ("I want to stay over at Billy's house!") but they're not yet able to reason it out in an adult way ("Why? You saw him yesterday." "Because I *do!*").

The still-changing frontal lobes also explain why adolescents are rarely paragons of subtlety. Teens are still learning to see the world from another person's perspective, and they lack the expertise to read other people's expressions. As a result, teens may be tactless, blurt out something inappropriate, or miss the nuances of speech. The rhetorical reprimand of a teacher, "Are you sure you want to do that?", may be met with an obnoxious-sounding, "Yes, I am!" Research shows that it is much more effective for teachers and parents to be unambiguous: "Please stop doing that."

WANT TO **GET ON BETTER WITH YOUR TEEN ALIEN**?

1
UNDERSTAND THEY CAN'T HELP IT—risk-taking and thrill-seeking are driven by their brain's overactive reward center.

2
USE STRAIGHTFORWARD LANGUAGE and avoid rhetorical or sarcastic retorts, which developing teenage brains can be poor at interpreting.

3
ALLOW THINKING TIME—while neuro-circuitry is being forged and refined, teens are fast to feel emotions and slower to make reasoned decisions.

JUDGING YOUTH IS NOTHING NEW

Writings reveal that the Ancient Greeks saw young people as having "bad manners, contempt for authority, disrespect to elders, and a love for chatter in place of exercise." Later, the philosopher Aristotle said of the "high-minded" youth that they "think they know everything and are quite sure of it."

And if you think that modern media are to blame for corrupting youth, then you join a long line of anxious adults. Enos Hitchcock, a Christian chaplain during the American Revolutionary War, said: "the free access which many young people have to romances, novels, and plays has poisoned the mind and corrupted the morals of many a promising youth." And if you believe an 1858 report in *Scientific American*, modern gaming may well be harmless compared to the "pernicious excitement" that comes from playing chess.

Some things just never change: perhaps it's best for us all to relax because, after all, your parents' generation said all those things about you, and you turned out just fine, didn't you?

Why Did I Take More Risks When I Was Younger?

If your bungee-jumping kit is gathering dust these days, you might wonder why leaping from a great height no longer appeals to you. The blame lies with your sensible brain.

Ask yourself: when were the best, most memorable days of your life? According to research, your most meaningful and vivid memories come from your adolescence, when your brain was drinking in life's experiences.

In the more adventurous adolescent years, a reward-seeking part of the brain called the nucleus accumbens is super-sensitive. Humans are driven by here-and-now rewards in their teen years more than at any other time in their lives. Dopamine-motivated desires are so powerful and the forward-thinking mind so immature that we are much more likely to be impulsive and

rash. Without the brakes of a fully operational frontal lobe, there is a tendency to "act first and think later."

As adults, we are less emotionally driven and dopamine-motivated because the analytical and planning parts of our brains have fully developed, allowing us to assess risks and make smarter choices accordingly.

Of course, many adults still take up thrill-seeking hobbies. They may have a gene that weakens the dopamine-throttling controls in the brain, meaning they get a bigger gush of feel-good dopamine when they drive fast, skydive, or snowboard the slopes.

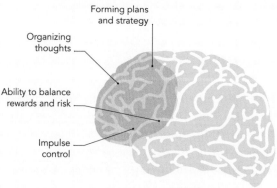

Forming plans and strategy

Organizing thoughts

Ability to balance rewards and risk

Impulse control

BRAIN

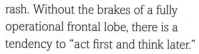

WORK IN PROGRESS
The so-called "responsible adult" part of your brain is called the prefrontal cortex, marked red in this image. This is where you assess thoughts and emotions and balance your desires and impulses against risk. During adolescence, this area rewires itself (see pages 118–119).

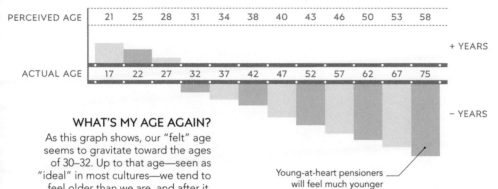

| PERCEIVED AGE | 21 | 25 | 28 | 31 | 34 | 38 | 40 | 43 | 46 | 50 | 53 | 58 |
| ACTUAL AGE | 17 | 22 | 27 | 32 | 37 | 42 | 47 | 52 | 57 | 62 | 67 | 75 |

+ YEARS

– YEARS

WHAT'S MY AGE AGAIN?

As this graph shows, our "felt" age seems to gravitate toward the ages of 30–32. Up to that age—seen as "ideal" in most cultures—we tend to feel older than we are, and after it, we see ourselves as younger, drifting ever further from reality as we age.

Young-at-heart pensioners will feel much younger than they really are

Why Do I Feel Younger Than My Real Age?

Almost all of us feel younger than we are in reality—yet more evidence of how poor we humans are at keeping track of time.

Research shows that we rarely feel the actual age we are (see above). This mismatch also explains why others seem to be getting younger. If we "feel" 40, but are actually much older, then a 25-year-oldpolice officer looks positively school age to us! Some researchers think that we unconsciously shift our mindset toward the age we want to be based on negative ideas about being "too old" or "too young." Incredibly, the rate at which our bodies undergo biological wear and tear appears to be slower nowadays, thanks to a global rise in quality of life—with fewer people smoking, improving health care, and better nutrition, people today are biologically about a year younger than an identically aged person two decades earlier. And even more incredibly, how old we feel seems to affect our health and how long we will live—with those who feel youngest on the inside likely to have fewer illnesses, better mental health, lower chances of dementia, and healthy bodies that will last well into old age.

Why Do Long-Past Events Seem So Recent to Me?

"But it feels like it was only yesterday!" When we can't believe how much time has passed since an event, we can blame a time-keeping glitch in our brains.

Think of a dramatic news event from a while ago and quickly guesstimate how long ago it happened. The chances are that you will underestimate just how many years have passed.

Whether it's movies you've seen, books you've read, family celebrations, or political upheavals, your memories of events that took place before a certain cutoff point will feel like they happened more recently due to a weird mental shortcut called the "telescoping effect." No one is sure whether this quirk is due to how your long-term memory organizes key events or whether it's a feature of how the brain ages, but telescoping has the effect of making recent events feel distant and distant events seem more recent.

The revelation that it has been 10 years since a famous celebrity died may make you feel suddenly old, but it can also trip you into thinking that everything from birthdays to natural disasters happen more often than they really do.

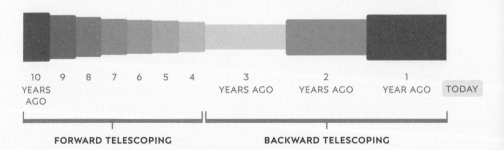

| 10 YEARS AGO | 9 | 8 | 7 | 6 | 5 | 4 | 3 YEARS AGO | 2 YEARS AGO | 1 YEAR AGO | TODAY |

FORWARD TELESCOPING   BACKWARD TELESCOPING

"WAS IT REALLY THAT LONG AGO?"

A quirk of the long-term memory, called the "telescoping effect," means that we perceive the three most recent years of our lives as lasting longer. The years before that seem to "bunch up"; events that took place a long time ago jump forward in our perception of time.

Why Are My Childhood Memories So Hazy?

At different stages of life, the brain has different priorities—some functions, such as storing memories, have to take a back seat in favor of more urgent jobs.

You almost certainly have no memories of your life before the age of three, and memories up to around age seven are probably patchy and vague. Throughout our earliest years, the hippocampus's cells are growing and in constant flux, making it difficult for strong memory pathways to establish. Early infant memories do form temporarily but are wiped at around age six, when memory circuits mature. The best efforts of memory-recovery "experts" can't reverse this childhood amnesia.

The early years are a critical time for how the brain develops. The procedural memory connections to and from the cerebellum and "habit hub" form first, enabling us to learn to talk, walk, and feed ourselves, before forming long-term memory stores. These are critical periods in early brain development devoted to procedural memory, emotions, and language; research shows that the human brain is far more able to learn at this time than at any other point in our lives.

So if you don't remember much from your childhood, take heart—it just means that your brain put all its energy into setting you up for the future.

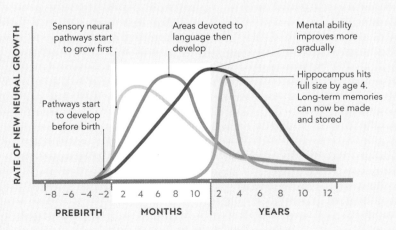

RATE OF NEW NEURAL GROWTH

Sensory neural pathways start to grow first

Areas devoted to language then develop

Mental ability improves more gradually

Hippocampus hits full size by age 4. Long-term memories can now be made and stored

Pathways start to develop before birth

PREBIRTH —8 —6 —4 —2

MONTHS 2 4 6 8 10

YEARS 2 4 6 8 10 12

CHILDISH BRAIN

When you were a young child, your brain's priority in the first year was learning how to speak, walk, and take in the world around you. The memory region, the hippocampus, isn't fully developed until the ages of 3–5.

Why Do I Remember Events Differently from Others?

After a disagreement, both parties can be adamant that their version of events is true. In reality, memory is fallible, and we are left grasping at straws.

The brain is simply not large enough to store the entire tsunami of experiences hitting us at every waking moment. When events—big or small—happen, they aren't taped onto a movie reel in your head. Rather, your brain is more like the photographer at a movie premier—quickly snapping those moments of the event that they deem worthy of saving. When you retell the event, these moments are pieced together and reconstructed, much like an inspired-by-true-events documentary.

The brain hates an incomplete story, so it can't help itself but to complete a fragmented memory by using its memory stores to bring sense to the uncertain haze.

If you're absolutely convinced by yourself or someone else that something happened in your past, then your memory circuitry may construct a "real" memory to fit this reality. In experiments where people were shown a photograph of themselves as a child in a hot-air balloon, about half said they could remember something of the trip. Only later was it revealed to them

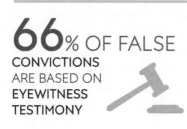

66% OF FALSE CONVICTIONS ARE BASED ON EYEWITNESS TESTIMONY

MISSING LINK

Your brain rarely stores a pristine, perfect snapshot of any event. It will fill in the blanks for you with a personalized touch, resulting in slightly different memories for everyone who witnessed a certain event.

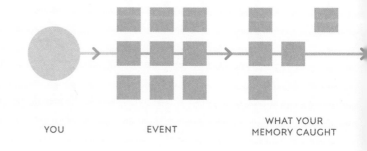

YOU   EVENT   WHAT YOUR MEMORY CAUGHT

that the photo was a fake, doctored to have their face superimposed.

Memories can be frustratingly incomplete and vague, but they nevertheless shape and mold your identity and unique personal story. Since highly emotional experiences are more likely to be remembered (see pages 132–133), these will influence how you might fill in certain gaps later. Your "documentary" will always have a highly personal slant.

If you're looking for something to back up a memory or claim, rely on hard evidence, such as texts or an unedited photo. But when it comes to who said what during an argument, it might be best to concede that because our memories are unreliable witnesses, the truth will always be somewhere in the middle.

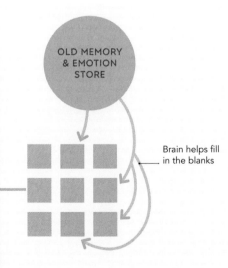

OLD MEMORY & EMOTION STORE

Brain helps fill in the blanks

SHOULD I TRUST MY MEMORY?

The shifting sands of our memories can cause problems and even lead to personal tragedy.

In 2015, US journalist and television presenter Brian Williams became a high-profile victim of the wobbly nature of the remembering mind, losing his job for falsely recounting a personal story. He had openly spoken about a terrifying experience during the 2003 Iraq War of being inside a military helicopter while it was shot at by rockets and forced to crash land.

Williams did indeed travel in a military helicopter, but, rather than being under fire himself, he had been told at the time of another aircraft ahead of them that had been forced into an emergency landing. Over the years, and possibly by melding his experiences with other news reports, his account morphed until, eventually, he became a passenger in the stricken helicopter. Williams had most likely unwittingly inserted false details into an actual event through its repeated retelling.

What Is *Déjà Vu,* and Should I Worry?

Neither a glitch in the Matrix nor a warning sign of failing memory, *déjà vu* is the result of your frontal lobe's obsessive tendency to connect dots that aren't there.

Most of us know the feeling: you arrive at a new place and have the distinct impression that you've been there before, or perhaps you are talking to a stranger and have the sense that you have already had the very same conversation. This is *déjà vu*, from the French "already seen," defined as a feeling of familiarity without an actual memory to anchor it to.

Your brain is continually screening your every sensation and thought, checking for familiar experiences so that it can anticipate what's going to happen next. When a sight, sound, or sensation is flagged as familiar, the hippocampus rifles through its store of long-term memories, like a librarian, to pull out a past similar experience. If the hippocampus draws a blank and the connection between the familiar feeling and a past memory cannot be made, then we are left with an uprooted feeling of familiarity—*déjà vu*.

This experience is most often linked to new places, so if you are a frequent traveler, you're likely to experience *déjà vu* more often. Sometimes, however, it seems that *déjà vu* has no foundation in

AN **AVERAGE**
25-YEAR-OLD EXPERIENCES
DÉJÀ VU AROUND
ONCE A MONTH

the real world but rather is a simple brain glitch, which occurs when neural pathways in the temporal lobes near the hippocampus spontaneously misfire. This is sometimes accompanied by the uncanny sense that you "knew" what was going to happen (although the science shows us that this belief is imagined).

Some scientists think this type of *déjà vu* occurs when an experience accidentally bypasses short-term memory storage and is filed directly into long-term memory stores, thus creating the sudden sensation that recent experience happened long ago.

Déjà vu is absolutely normal and most common in early adulthood, when the brain is at its busiest; children and the elderly experience far fewer episodes.

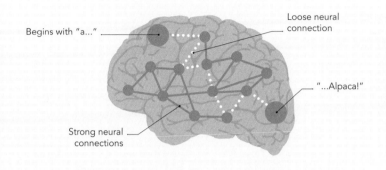

Begins with "a..."

Loose neural connection

Strong neural connections

"...Alpaca!"

THE MISSING LINK
Your brain is a matted
spider's web of neural
connections, some of
them much stronger
than others. Connections
are weaker between
distantly related
topics—the link is there;
it just needs some
nudging to reignite it.

What Is That "On-the-Tip-of-My-Tongue" Feeling?

You're trying to remember a quiz answer, but it's as if your tires are spinning in snow. This frustrating memory hiccup is due to weak brain connections about unfamiliar topics.

"What's the name of the animal that's related to the llama and begins with 'a'?" You *know* what it's called, but because it's been ages since you visited a farm, the neural connection between the name and the clue is weak. Names, places, numbers, and facts are called semantic memories and are far weaker than our memories of stories and real experiences. Your brain is trying to find the route back to this key fact, but the trail of bread crumbs has become messy.

When you have had a "tip-of-the-tongue" moment for a name once, you're actually more likely to have the same feeling next time. The tortuous reremembering journey is likely to be repeated each time you try to remember the name, unless you can form new, fresh associations to your existing pool of knowledge.

It's at these times when a relaxed mind can unlock these stuck facts. New connections are both formed and found more freely when the mind is in its wandering "default mode network". The chances are you'll be lying in bed one evening, and the penny-dropping moment comes:
"I've got it—alpaca!"

Why Do I Sometimes Forget Why I Came into the Room?

When you enter a room for a reason but then can't for the life of you remember why, you're experiencing an eerie feature of the mind's energy-saving economy.

The "doorway effect" is the term used for when parts of your short-term memory get wiped clean whenever you enter a new location—even if it's a virtual one.

Your "working memory" is the part of your short-term memory circuitry that holds information for the here and now. It can hold between only three and seven different things at a time. Entering a new location tells the brain the situation has changed and that those chunks of information are no longer relevant, so it's safe to discard them to make room for new things. It's a healthy way for the brain to make the most efficient use of your limited temporary memory.

The doorway effect happens just as often in the young and old so needn't cause you to fret that your memory is failing. Return to the original room or retrace your steps mentally, and you will often recall or figure out the thought process that led you here.

THE DOORWAY EFFECT
Entering a new room often tells the brain to start afresh to free up space for new information. The more tasks you are trying to remember, the more likely it is that you will be at the mercy of the doorway effect.

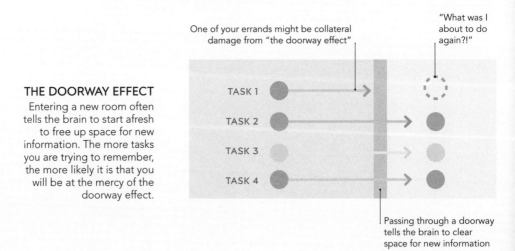

One of your errands might be collateral damage from "the doorway effect"

"What was I about to do again?!"

TASK 1
TASK 2
TASK 3
TASK 4

Passing through a doorway tells the brain to clear space for new information

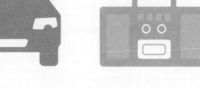

Why Can I Remember Faces Better Than Names?

That person looks so familiar, but you just can't think of their name. Don't be embarrassed—your brain's got an unfair advantage at remembering faces over names.

A large part of the visual brain is devoted to seeing faces. Picking out a face amid an out-of-focus haze is a matter of survival: soon after birth, we must find our mother's face—the source of nourishment and our first protector. Research shows that just a few hours after birth, a baby can spot facial features even if there is no actual face—just a curved line with two dots above it.

This preprogrammed preference for spotting possible faces is carried throughout our lives. Our social ancestors needed it to recognize friends, cooperate for survival, and distinguish potential rivals. Our visual processing centers, toward the back of the brain, have a sophisticated "facial vocabulary," capable of storing around 10,000 faces. You are far less likely to recall a name, however, because your brain stores them separately as semantic memories with no obvious link to what they look like.

Memories are more likely to be stored long term if they also carry an emotional attachment; unless you had a meaningful exchange with someone, you're likely to have long forgotten their name but still remember their face if you spot them a few months later.

Why Can I Still Remember Skills, Even Years Later?

When it comes to learned skills, especially those involving repeated movements, your brain's most primal regions are like a memory-foam mattress.

Ten, 20, 30, or more years may have passed since you last mounted your childhood BMX (complete with tassels), but you haven't forgotten how to ride. Like writing, swimming, driving, or typing on a keyboard, the ability stays with you, long after the hours of learning are forgotten. Sometimes called "muscle memory" (correctly termed procedural memory), muscles themselves have little to do with it.

Rather, these skills are stored in the cerebellum, far from your conscious memories of events. A large wrinkled

region tucked under the back of the brain, the cerebellum is under the orchestration of a curved tadpole-shaped structure in the middle of the brain called the basal ganglia.

With each attempt at a skill, slowly but surely, a path of neural connections forms in the brain. Through repetition and practice, these abilities build a well-trodden walkway deep inside your brain's circuitry. The weeds of time are slow to obscure this path, so you will be able to retrace your steps and get back into the saddle well into your old

SHARP FOCUS

The brain undergoes three different stages when learning a new skill, such as playing the piano. Neural pathways grow in number with time, and the pathways remain fairly strong over many years.

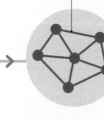

Weak neural pathways

Strong neural pathways

Neural pathways retain most of their strength

Neural pathways for procedural memory form in cerebellum

FIRST FEW CLASSES

ACCOMPLISHED PIANIST

PICKING UP AFTER A FEW YEARS

age, even if you're a bit rusty. It takes an estimated 20 hours of deliberate, focused practice to gain basic skills in a new hobby. Expert craftspeople and athletes take somewhere in the region of 10,000 hours firming up brain pathways before they reach the top of their game.

It's not only the highly skilled who rely on procedural memory; most of what you do every day is executed on "autopilot," such as brushing your teeth or getting dressed. These tasks require

IT TAKES AROUND

25,000

HOURS OF PRACTICE FOR A **CLASSICAL MUSICIAN** TO REACH THE **PEAK** OF THEIR **SKILLS**

very little conscious thought because they are run via the basal ganglia rather than being under the direct control of the frontal, decision-making brain regions, which are free to focus on other things. If we didn't have these programs, we would have to concentrate every time we tie our shoelaces.

These "unthinking" skills become so well established that they actually outperform our conscious brain's ability for that task. When we try to think too much about something we're good at, we can "choke," which has been many an athlete's undoing on the day of the big event.

THE UNFORGETTABLE BRAIN OF MOLAISON

In 1953, pioneering neurosurgeon Dr. William Scoville performed neurosurgery on Henry Molaison. Henry was alert but anesthetized as his skull was opened and portions of his brain removed. At the time, no one knew what the hippocampus did, but Dr. Scoville had a misguided hunch that this structure was the reason for the epilepsy that had plagued Henry. Sadly, the operation left the 27-year-old unable to ever make a new conscious memory.

Henry's epilepsy mercifully settled, and his personality and intellect were unaffected, but he would forget events after a few minutes. Incredibly, though, his "habit hub" (basal ganglia) and procedural memory circuitry were intact. He was able to learn new skills even though he instantly forgot how he had learned them.

Through studying Henry's brain, scientists found that our regular memory and our "muscle" memory are stored in separate areas. From what we've learned from his brain, patients suffering memory loss can be rehabilitated faster by teaching them new techniques and skills.

How Can I Improve My Memory?

Some people are gifted with an elephant-like memory, others with a Dory-like recall. The key to a better memory is to repeat, repeat, repeat, with a touch of emotion.

The photographer of the "documentary" that is your life story is an inch-long, slug-shaped region in the brain called the hippocampus, nestled within the head of the coiling snake of the emotional limbic circuit. Your emotions—good and bad—are the gatekeeper of what makes it in and what gets left on the cutting-room floor. You won't remember what you ate for breakfast last Wednesday because it wasn't exciting, but if your lover got down on one knee to propose to you that morning, the fact you were eating a bowl of oatmeal at the time will be forever remembered, as clear as day.

That's why dry lectures, dreary news bulletins, and boring books leave your head almost as soon as they are over. You'll forget an arbitrary fact—such as 1769 being the year French ruler Napoleon Bonaparte was born—by the time you turn the page because it has no significance to you. However, if you love all things locomotive, then you may have noted to yourself that this was the same year that the steam engine was invented, making Napoleon's birthday easier to remember. The frontal lobe pathways for new memories and information will sprout from your established memory patterns, much like a new branch budding from an old grape vine.

Crucially, memories are packaged into

WANT A **SUPER-MEMORY**?

1
KEEP A DIARY to record memories as soon as possible after the event, before they are contaminated by emotions or misty recollections.

2
TELL STORIES, because repeating anecdotes to others will help form very strong memories by tying positive emotions to them, making the memory more likely to stick in your long-term stores.

3
CREATE MIND MAPS to make visual connections between pieces of information that you want to learn. The more connections you make within a topic, the more likely you'll retain information.

4
TRY RHYMES to create associations between letters or numbers and physical objects. (One = bread bun, Two = leather shoe, Three = oak tree, etc.)

long-term storage only once you have brought them back to mind at least once. Everyone loves stories—they are the linchpin of our understanding of the world, and we often entertain friends with fond memories that begin with "remember the time when ..." and reminisce with family over tales from childhood. Each time you recall the memory, its neural pathways become strengthened and thickened and more likely to weather the passage of time.

AFTER SIX MONTHS, AROUND
25% OF DETAILS OF AN EVENT MAY BE **REPLACED** WITH **FABRICATED** **DETAILS**

Your memory is at its worst when your body clock is slumping. For most of us, this will be the late afternoon and early evening; however, for night owls this is the morning.

Even though memories are famously fallible (see pages 124–125), you can look to the box to the left for tips and tricks on how to improve your everyday recall. The tips might even help you study for an exam or remember key information at work.

WHEN MEMORIES GO WRONG

In extreme events—such as a violent assault, abuse, or life-threatening accident—memories can be kept in such harsh focus that they bubble to the surface and haunt us for years. They become part of post-traumatic stress disorder (PTSD), the hallmarks of which are vivid and distressing flashbacks, nightmares, and bouts of anxiety.

For many years, "debriefing" was routinely offered to people involved in a traumatic event, but this process of forced reliving of the ordeal soon after the event causes the emotional intensity of the memory to be magnified, worsening symptoms.

Today, PTSD is treated with trauma-tailored cognitive-behavioral therapy to understand the triggers and effectively process what happened so that the memories are less intense and less likely to resurface.

Should I Always Believe What I See?

When we look around us, the world appears as a crisp, full-color, wide-screen video. But in fact, most of what you see is just a figment of your imagination.

In 2015, a photo of a dress shared on social media famously split the world in two: half of us saw a white and gold dress, with the other half convinced it was blue and black. How could that be possible? The answer lies in the limitations of what we're capable of seeing. Our brains fill in the gaps for us.

Clear color vision comes from a tiny 0.3 mm patch on the back of the eye, called the fovea, where light from the center of your gaze is focused. Everything outside of this is fuzzy and colorless. Suppose you are jogging, wind in your hair, down a wooded track, enjoying the lush green trees lining the path on both sides. In fact, nearly all of the vibrant leafy vista is a black-and-white blur that your brain has conjured into clear, verdant color, based on what it received when you last looked directly at the view.

Turning the two, incomplete blurry images received from each eye into a convincing three-dimensional world calls for a lot of brain cells to do a lot of hard work. Electrical impulses from the back of your eyes hurtle through the brain to the visual cortex, which systematically analyzes what we see for shapes, colors, and familiar features, such as figures or faces.

SHARP-EYED? THINK AGAIN!

If you're holding this book at arm's length away from you, your brain interprets everything to be in clear focus. But in fact, the only thing that your eyes can really focus on is the fingernail-sized shape in the middle of your vision—represented by an in-focus green block here. Everything else gets more blurry and colorless the farther away from the green block you get.

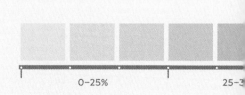

0–25%　　　　　25–3

At each staging post on the image's journey, the brain needs to make assumptions and shortcuts, and we all have these "cheat sheets."

Back to the great dress controversy. Subsequent studies showed that the divided opinions were down to the assumptions our brains made when we first saw the image. If your brain assumes the image was lit by a camera flash from the front, then the dress appears to be blue and black; whereas if your split-second judgment decides it was lit by a window behind the dress, it's unmistakably white and gold to you. (If the controversy passed you by, search online for "the dress" to make your own mind up.) Your initial assumptions will stick—it's almost impossible to see the dress how the other 50 percent do.

0.3
SECONDS—THE TIME IT TAKES FOR THE BRAIN TO PROCESS WHAT WE SEE

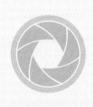

Like your unreliable memory (see pages 124–125), be aware that your vision can be just as untrustworthy. The mind is a finely tuned guessing machine, built on a lifetime of experiences. However, when it comes down to giving an eye-witness account, keep in mind that your best guess is often inaccurate if you didn't get a good, straight-on view.

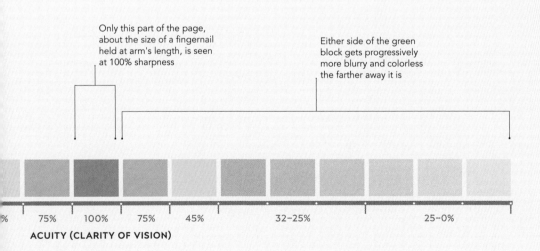

Only this part of the page, about the size of a fingernail held at arm's length, is seen at 100% sharpness

Either side of the green block gets progressively more blurry and colorless the farther away it is

| % | 75% | 100% | 75% | 45% | | 32–25% | | 25–0% |

ACUITY (CLARITY OF VISION)

Is It True We Use Only 10 Percent of Our Brains?

The notion that there are vast, untapped regions of our brains waiting to be unlocked is persistent—and utter nonsense. We use every single brain cell.

The idea that we use only a fraction of our brain power was first put forward by psychologists in the late 1800s. It's been disproved countless times, but we hold on to this myth because it speaks to our longing to be better, smarter people—harness this hidden promise, and maybe we would even be able to outwit Einstein.

Weighing in at just 3 lb (1.4 kg), the brain contains around 100 billion neurons, each relaying electrically powered impulses and communicating via chemical signals with up to 1,000 of its neighbors. Like minute cogs in a vast machine, each cell has a job to do.

However, the brain is more than a warehouse-sized supercomputer. Unlike digital machines, it is constantly in flux,

IT WOULD TAKE
1 MILLION
INTERCONNECTED PROCESSORS TO MIMIC **JUST 1%** OF THE SCALE OF THE **HUMAN BRAIN**

with new connections forming every second. It offers us unimaginable potential to change and learn. No urban myths required.

BUSY BRAIN

Brain scans show that no part of the brain lies unused. Parts of our brains are used at different times, depending on what we're doing (see page 70).

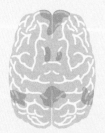
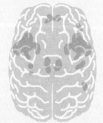
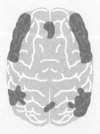

"WANDERING" NETWORK   "WATCHING" NETWORK   "CONCENTRATION" NETWORK

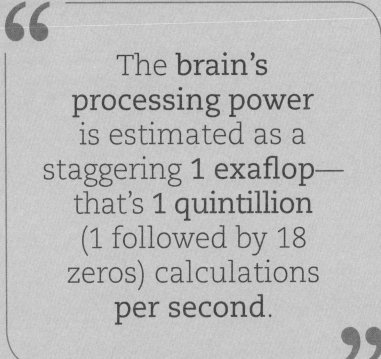

"
The **brain's
processing power**
is estimated as a
staggering **1 exaflop**—
that's **1 quintillion**
(1 followed by 18
zeros) calculations
per second.
"

Can I Raise My IQ?

We revere intelligence and award "smart" people with a high IQ score, but are we really born with our intelligence, and can we actually learn to be smarter?

The IQ (intelligence quotient) score is an internationally accepted measure of total brain power, calculated via a series of tests. These tests usually involve math, spotting patterns, and logic—so if your forte lies in practical problem solving, negotiating with others, or creativity, the chances are you won't excel at an IQ test.

Intelligence has no clear definition. Like beauty or personality, it's relatively subjective, and this is one reason IQ scores are problematic.

Another issue is that IQ tests have historically been created by (mostly) men in Europe and North America— and are skewed in favor of people from Western culture. Someone from a community that values storytelling, for example, may have great verbal reasoning and memory, yet their overall IQ score might be low because they flopped on the number puzzles.

So although scientists have worked hard to make tests reliable and relevant across cultures, IQ tests have a limited

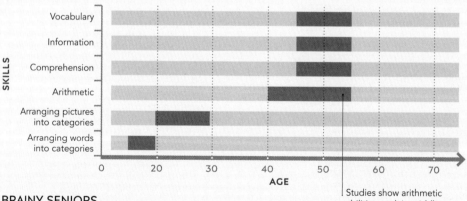

Studies show arithmetic abilities peak in middle age

BRAINY SENIORS

Your brain will mature as you get older, and you will reach your peak at certain skills later in your life. For example, you might struggle with mental arithmetic when you're 25—then by the time you're 50, sums become a breeze.

KEY

■ Peak activity

use. For mentally taxing jobs, such as programming, a test is an effective barometer for picking the best recruit. However, if we were patients given the choice between a 22-year-old novice surgeon with a genius IQ and a 55-year-old expert with countless successful operations under their belt, we all know who we would rather cut us open.

Experience, knowledge, social skills, drive, and conscientiousness—all of which could all be considered intelligence—are not accounted for in the conventional IQ test. Even though young adults tend to get the best overall IQ scores, just like a fine wine, many of our abilities continue to improve with age.

Good IQ score or not, everyone can improve their cognitive powers, regardless of their age, schooling, and past experience. Don't be sold on quick fixes—brain training games and programs will help you get better at those games and tasks but rarely translate into any practical thinking powers. To get really good at something—be it memorizing place names, coding software, or crafting musical compositions—you'll need to practice that particular skill for many hours (see pages 130–131).

IQ'S FASCIST HISTORY

The first intelligence tests were devised by French psychologist Alfred Binet in the early 1900s as a benevolent way to find the least able children who needed special schooling. A strong believer in the idea that intellectual prowess was not set in stone and could be improved with teaching, practice, and discipline, Binet insisted that intelligence tests should never be used "for ranking [people] according to mental worth."

Soon after his death in 1911, however, Binet's test, later named "IQ" tests, were seized by scientists in the eugenics movement who reformulated it for adults, labeling those who scored poorly as "feeble-minded" or "degenerate." In the early 1900s, 30 US states passed laws that meant low-scoring people could be forcibly sterilized. By the middle of the 20th century, around 60,000 people had been sterilized against their will.

Adolf Hitler also espoused the IQ test and created his own stylized version. Hundreds of thousands of low-scoring people were duly sterilized or executed in Nazi Germany.

How Can I Avoid Buying Things I Don't Need?

If your lunchtime shopping errand turns into a spree, it may be down to smart retailers exploiting your emotions. Most of your shopping decisions aren't based on rational thought.

You probably think you're a smart shopper, but when you buy something new, you're first satisfying your unthinking, emotional mind. Only afterward, perhaps on your way home, do you employ logical thinking to justify why you made the best, most reasonable choice.

Store policies such as try-before-you-buy seem to appeal to our common sense; they offer us the chance to make sure we are spending money on something that fits our requirements. This is a half-truth; the ploy is to make us feel a sense of ownership over the

95% OF **SHOPPING DECISIONS** ARE BASED ON **EMOTIONS**, NOT LOGIC

product. Termed the "endowment effect," you won't want to give the product back because your mind sees it as belonging to you. Most powerful with physical objects, the effect also applies to online subscriptions and digital purchases. Another aspect of the endowment effect is that we invariably put an inflated price tag on items we own—for instance, you will think that a beautiful lamp that cost you $10 is worth double that amount to a stranger who wants to buy it from you.

This train of thought can push you into making foolish decisions; for instance, stock market investors typically hold on to their shares for too long after their value has slumped, refusing to believe that they aren't worth keeping.

WANT TO GIVE YOUR **BANK ACCOUNT A BREAK?**

1

AVOID FREE TRIALS, because when you start to feel like the product is yours, the endowment effect may take hold.

2

REMEMBER THAT it's statistically unlikely you will return a high value item, such as a car, bed, or smartphone.

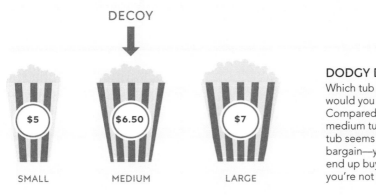

DECOY

$5 — SMALL
$6.50 — MEDIUM
$7 — LARGE

DODGY DECOYS
Which tub of popcorn would you choose? Compared to the medium tub, the large tub seems like a bargain—you might end up buying it even if you're not that hungry!

Why Can I Never Find the Best Bargains?

Free samples and reduced prices don't always mean saving money—they can be part of a strategy to make you feel good enough to spend, spend, spend.

If you want to hack a person's good sense, just try offering them something for nothing. Like moths to a flame, shoppers swarm for free gifts, as if they had left their brains at the door.

We tend to feel indebted to anyone who gives us a gift. It's a psychological law of the jungle known as "reciprocity." Someone offers you something and you'll be inclined to give something in return (for example, by actually paying for the product you've just tasted or been given a sample of).

This tit-for-tat reciprocity is the social glue that keeps communities together:

monkeys groom each other; birds guard their neighbors' nests out of an ancient public spirit. Reciprocity can be used for long-term gain, too; restaurant owners who give patrons a complementary starter or free drink at the end of the meal do so knowing it's likely they will be rewarded with a five-star review and a loyal customer.

Our love of a bargain can also be exploited by placing vastly overpriced "decoy" items among more normal-priced ones. By comparison, the item with a "normal" price looks like a true bargain, so we eagerly snap it up.

How Can I Shop Most Effectively?

There are many psychological tricks that stores and supermarkets employ to get you to spend money. Know how to spot them so that you can hold on to your cash.

Stores have long been priming us with the subliminal message that more is always better. Take shopping baskets—these were once small enough to tuck under one arm but have grown larger and larger. Today's wheeled, "small" baskets with extendable handles are about the same size as the largest shopping carts available in the 1930s.

Some stores employ mazelike layouts—customers are obliged to browse, as it's practically impossible to dash in just to pick up a specific item. The path leads through numerous showrooms, all displaying tempting low-cost items. Each different area we enter resets our short-term memory because of the doorway effect, helping

Colors influence shopping habits— products with bright yellow or red price tags sell more

The most expensive, branded products are placed just below eye level

The cheapest products are usually farthest from the entrance, forcing you to walk past other products

The hidden bargains can often be found by hunting on the lowest or highest shelves

ALL'S FAIR IN SHOPPING AND WAR

Stores are set up to maximize profit, which means taking every opportunity to get customers to buy more.

us forget what we were originally looking for (see page 128). The winding layout also encourages us to pick up products on impulse, as we worry we might not be able to find them again! Another trick on similar lines is to constantly change the layout of the store, so customers have to look for their favorite items, passing other tempting products on the way.

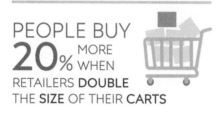

PEOPLE BUY
20% MORE WHEN
RETAILERS **DOUBLE**
THE **SIZE** OF THEIR **CARTS**

WANT TO BE A **SAVVY SHOPPER?**

1

WRITE A SHOPPING LIST as a countermeasure to the doorway effect. Trying to remember what you came for makes you vulnerable to distraction and impulse buying.

2

USE A HAND BASKET if you can—you won't be tempted to fill a large cart, you'll be limited by what you can physically carry, and so you'll buy only what you need.

3

DON'T RUSH—when we are under pressure of time, we take mental shortcuts that make rash decisions more likely.

4

LISTEN TO MUSIC or a podcast on headphones to blot out the store's musical attempts to alter your mood or your shopping pace.

Shelves may be part-filled, to make a product seem sought after (the "scarcity effect")

On a price tag, the digit we notice most is the first one—this "left digit bias" means we assess $49.99 as much cheaper than $50

$49.99

Slow music makes shoppers linger; upbeat music makes shoppers move and choose faster

Sweets are placed at the eye level of a child

Larger carts tempt customers to fill them

Is It Cheaper to Shop Online?

You might think you can avoid retailers' tricks by surfing the net and bagging the best deals, but the online marketplace has its pitfalls, too.

For most of human history, we have haggled in the marketplace over the price of almost everything, from camels to corsets. The final price depended on largely the relationship between seller and shopper.

Fixed prices didn't come until much later and were introduced in an effort to make shopping fairer for all.

71% OF SHOPPERS
THINK THEY GET A **BETTER DEAL** **ONLINE** THAN IN A PHYSICAL STORE

WANT TO WIN AT ONLINE SHOPPING?

1

TAKE "PRICE REDUCTIONS" with a pinch of salt—the old prices may have been conjured out of thin air. There are few laws that stop online retailers from doing this.

2

SIGN UP TO AUTOMATIC ALERTS from websites or apps that track the prices of flights, food, and books and update you when rates take a plunge.

3

BEWARE OF "ONLY TWO LEFT!" notifications—fear of missing out (the "scarcity effect") might prompt you to rush to the checkout, but often the claims are not true.

Now, online shopping, with its artificial intelligence and algorithms, has brought variable pricing back to the mainstream—although this time around, shoppers are kept in the dark. Algorithms are used to predict demand, and retailers adjust their prices accordingly. Some cold-drink vending machines, for example, are now programmed to charge more on hot days, because you'll be willing to cough up more cash when you're parched.

The return to fluctuating prices doesn't have to be bad news for consumers, however; you just need to be wise to the invisible market forces to bag the bargains.

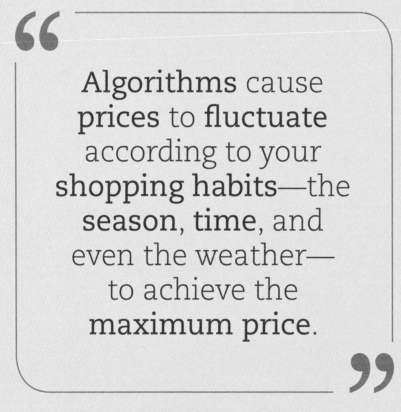

"
Algorithms cause prices to fluctuate according to your shopping habits—the season, time, and even the weather— to achieve the maximum price.
"

EVENING

Throwing off the weighty shackles of the afternoon fug, evening brings a second dawn to our body. Our internal machinery explodes into life once again, and buzzing brain networks rediscover their morning clarity and efficiency. Under the starter's orders of the body clock, limbs are loosened and creative juices flow. Socializing becomes smoother, and it's time to savor all that is good in life....

Why Is It Hard to Motivate Myself to Exercise?

Regular exercise keeps brain and body well oiled, yet for many of us, the promise of a healthier, happier life isn't enough to free us from the pull of the couch.

Running on a treadmill, going nowhere, endlessly pounding and staring at the same wall—it can seem like cruel torture, and that's because it originally was. Long before gyms, in the 1800s, treadmills started out as a punishment for troublesome prison inmates.

Criminal or not, if you consider yourself an exercise sluggard, then it may be in part due to your genes.

YOUR GENES INFLUENCE HOW MUCH YOU ENJOY EXERCISE BY UP TO 37%

We think we are masters of our own destiny, yet around half of your personality and temperament—including whether you enjoy or fear the treadmill—is inherited from your parents through DNA. Your reluctance to exercise may be partly due to a series of "laziness genes"—strips of DNA code that control the release of endorphins into the brain. These are the chemicals responsible for natural "highs" people experience during exercise (see page 157). To put it simply, you'll get less of an "exercise buzz" than others do.

You might find yourself avoiding workouts because the first few minutes of exercise feels like wading through quicksand, even for elite athletes. It takes a while for your lungs and muscles to respond fully to the sudden demands made on them. Until then, every step is a mountain, so go easy on yourself and don't give up.

Your arms and legs might also feel tingly at first—this is because tiny blood vessels under your skin, which were squashed flat while you were lounging about on the sofa, are suddenly blasted open by a flood of warm blood. Nerve receptors send signals to your brain, which temporarily misinterprets the gush as an uncomfortable tingle.

To help you get motivated, it may also be useful to know your chronotype (see pages 22–23) so that you can plan exercise for when your energy levels are highest. Also, if you eat the right food before a workout (see page 152), you can ensure that you're off to the best start possible.

30
SECONDS

When you start exercising, your newly flexing muscles rely on immediate stores of sugar (glycogen) for fuel. They're starved of the oxygen they need to keep going, so they quickly become clogged with acidic waste. They feel sluggish—it's hard to keep moving

1:30
MINUTES

It takes another minute or so before your muscles are suffused with enough oxygen-carrying blood for strong, steady contractions

3:00
MINUTES

Your lungs are beginning to fully expand, to give them maximum oxygen-sucking powers. Your body now relies on fuel stores from the liver (see pages 164–165)

5:00
MINUTES

Your body is now "primed," in sports-science terms, and will stay exercise-ready for up to 45 minutes, even if you take a break between warm-up and workout

FULLY PRIMED, YOUR LUNGS
CAN DELIVER UP TO
8 TIMES MORE OXYGEN TO THE HEART

BODY'S READINESS FOR EXERCISE

TIME

CLIMBING THE MOUNTAIN

For the first five or so minutes of exercise, your body is demanding energy more quickly than your lungs can provide oxygen to make it. Once your body is primed after about five minutes, it flips the biological switch to "aerobic" mode—now you're efficiently converting oxygen into fuel for your muscles, enabling you to train for endurance exercise effectively.

When Should I Exercise?

Your body is like a huge locomotive that takes an age to reach top speed. Leaving exercise until your body is ready means a better workout and fewer injuries.

Morning workouts are unquestionably good for you, your mood, and your concentration, and even help improve academic performance. However, this is the time for gentle exercise; if you push muscles beyond their capacity, they are liable to damage, resulting in tiny rips that cause soreness and injury. Save serious workouts for the afternoon when your body is at its peak. Also, avoid exercising too late in the evening—workouts raise your temperature, counteracting the natural lowering of your body temperature, which readies you for sleep.

Physical performance worsens during hot spells; exercise may feel easier to

BETWEEN **4PM** AND **8PM**, YOUR **PERFORMANCE** MAY BE BOOSTED BY **25**% COMPARED TO THE MORNING

start with, but you will tire much more quickly. On average, you'll probably do best at 65–68°F (18–20°C). Prolonged, vigorous physical exertion is best left for much cooler days—between 41–50°F (5–10°C)—and this may be why running on the treadmill in an air-conditioned gym can feel easier than pounding the pavement in summer.

PUSH IT BACK

Most people hit their physical prime about nine hours after they naturally wake; morning larks may take less time because they wake earlier, while night owls can take a bit longer since they usually wake later.

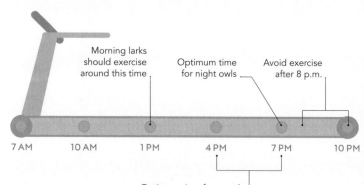

Morning larks should exercise around this time

Optimum time for night owls

Avoid exercise after 8 p.m.

7 AM   10 AM   1 PM   4 PM   7 PM   10 PM

Optimum time for people with average body clock

"

As the **day progresses** and your slowly digesting **breakfast replenishes** the **body's** easy-access **fuel stores**, so your **physical abilities** will **improve**.

"

What and When Should I Eat Before Exercise?

Exercise conflicts with the smooth running of the digestive system, so manage your nutrition and portion sizes the closer you get to your workout time.

Good nutrition and a varied diet is undeniably important for building fitness and strength. Food gives your body the fuel and building blocks to repair and restore after a workout. Digestion is slowed when exercising, so time meals carefully (see below). Any food eaten within an hour of setting off should ideally be an easily-digested carbohydrate snack or drink, which can give a final top up of fuel.

WHAT SHOULD I EAT?

- **Whole grain** bread, rice, or potatoes contain carbohydrates to top up your muscle and liver energy stores.
- **Meat, fish, eggs, and pulses** have protein that supplies amino acids for repairing and building muscles and other tissues damaged during exercise.
- **Oily fish and nuts** contain fats that give even longer-lasting energy than carbohydrates. Fats slam the brakes on digestion, though, so avoid them immediately before vigorous exercise.
- **Minimally processed foods** tend to be high in vitamins, minerals, and nutrients, which help your body repair itself after exercise.

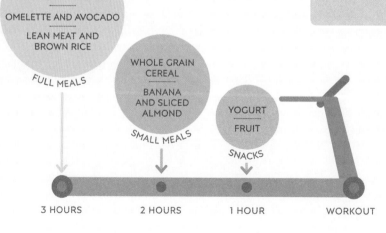

WHOLE GRAIN BREAD SANDWICH AND SALAD
—
OMELETTE AND AVOCADO
—
LEAN MEAT AND BROWN RICE

FULL MEALS

WHOLE GRAIN CEREAL
—
BANANA AND SLICED ALMOND

SMALL MEALS

YOGURT
—
FRUIT

SNACKS

3 HOURS   2 HOURS   1 HOUR   WORKOUT

PLAN AHEAD

Ideally, you should eat a full meal around three hours before a workout—any later and you risk cramps, indigestion, or heartburn. As you get nearer to the starting blocks, nourishment should get simpler, smaller, and easier to digest.

When Should I Eat After Exercise?

Is there really a 30-minute "window of opportunity" after exercise when your body sucks up nutrients like a dry sponge?

Many gym-goers worry that if they miss the "golden window" after exercise, they lose the chance to reap the rewards of their workout. In reality, there is a six-hour period during which fatigued muscle fibers need protein to help them repair after exercise. It also takes an hour and a half for most of the protein you have swallowed to break down into amino acids, enter the bloodstream, and reach muscle fibers. So relax; there's plenty of time for protein. However, a smaller window applies to carbs: easy-access glycogen stores in the muscles are refilled twice as quickly after exercise compared to two hours later. This may be useful if you're about to do more exercise, but if not, then eating a proper meal later in the day will fully replenish muscles.

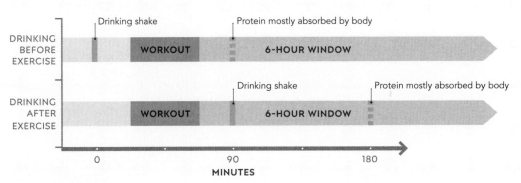

TAKE YOUR TIME

So when should you drink your protein shake? The truth is, it takes around 90 minutes for most of the protein to be absorbed, so you can slurp the shake before or after your workout and still get the full nutritional benefit.

Does Stretching Prevent Injury?

For weekend warriors and elite athletes alike, stretching is seen as a workout essential. The science behind it, however, turns out to be rather shaky.

Research says stretching before exercise doesn't prevent soreness, reduce injury, or improve performance. Furthermore, static stretching—where you hold a fixed pose for a few seconds—will inflict microscopic tears in your muscles, making you weaker and setting you up for injury. On the other hand, dynamic stretching—where you move your limbs and body around—doesn't harm your muscles.

Stretching *after* exercise can be useful, however. If you're looking for the flexibility to touch your toes, do the splits, or bend like a ballerina, then regular postexercise stretching can lengthen muscles and tendons, making your body more supple. However, some muscles simply can't be lengthened—attempting to force these muscles beyond their limited range can cause painful, long-term damage. Postexercise static stretching can help relax muscles and knock the edge off aches the next day—although it lowers soreness only by a measly 1 to 4 percent on average.

Even though stretching isn't all it's cracked up to be, it pays to ease off the gas slowly at the end of a workout. Gently spinning your legs on the bike after spin class or slowly jogging after a long run are the order of the day, reducing next-day soreness better than simply stretching would. If the workout has been particularly brutal, then a professional sports massage will help. Long seen by scientists as feeling nice but pointless, research now shows that massages, if conducted by a professional, can speed muscle recovery, reduce injury, and ease stiffness.

OTHER POSTEXERCISE RECOVERY RITUALS

1

DO SOME LIGHT EXERCISE to ease symptoms of muscle soreness, especially after running or cycling.

2

SCHEDULE IN REST DAYS where you do no exercise at all so that your body can repair muscles and recover fully.

How Can I Avoid Getting a Stitch?

Scientists call a stitch event-related transient abdominal pain (ETAP). Although there are some clues to go on, the jury is still out on what causes that strange, jabbing pain.

Often, a stitch—that agonizing pain just beneath the ribs—happens during bouncing activities, such as jogging and horse riding. This has led some scientists to theorize that stitches are caused by ligaments attached to your internal organs being strained from repeated jolts.

Another theory is that the up-down internal roller coaster may be stemming the blood supply to your diaphragm (the tough sheet of muscle

DURING A **MARATHON**,
ONE IN FIVE
ENTRANTS WILL **SUFFER** A **STITCH** AT SOME POINT

at the bottom of the chest that tugs down to inflate your lungs when you breathe in), causing it to cramp.

You're also more likely to get a stitch when exercising right after eating a meal or slurping a sugary drink—leading to yet another theory that the pain stems from cramping of the intestines or lack of blood to the guts.

Although elite athletes are not immune from side stitches, generally, the fitter you are, the less likely it is that you'll suffer them. It's not easy to avoid them—but there are some steps you can take to keep them at bay. And if a stitch does hit, ease up and wait until it passes.

WANT TO AVOID THOSE **PESKY STITCHES?**

1

START EXERCISE SLOWLY and pace yourself. A stitch is more likely to happen if you suddenly exert yourself.

2

AVOID EATING and drinking very sugary drinks just before exercise (sports drinks are usually fine).

3

KEEP AN UPRIGHT POSTURE so that you don't cramp your diaphragm or intestines.

What's the Best Exercise for a Healthy Heart?

Pounding away for hours on the treadmill is good for you, but it doesn't give your heart a thorough workout—quick, high-intensity sessions do that best.

Exercise is good for us because it puts a strain on the body, prompting it to toughen up for the next punishment. A violinist knows that the skin on their fingertips gets thicker and tougher after several weeks' practice, and so it is with exercise—the heart beats harder, lungs inflate more, and blood flows more smoothly around the body.

Cardio (short for "cardiovascular") exercise specifically targets these body systems. What you might think of as cardio exercises—running or swimming—certainly get your heart pounding and lungs working, but this kind of activity is actually better at strengthening your endurance muscles so they can work for longer.

Instead, what's best for your heart is short bursts of very vigorous, gasping-with-all-you've-got exercise, such as high-intensity interval training (HIIT). Putting your heart and lungs under blasts of intense strain, as if you were a cheetah suddenly chasing a gazelle after a day lounging in the sun, heightens the body's repairing and strengthening responses. These exercises will lower levels of artery-clogging cholesterol and protect you against diabetes, and you'll receive a particularly huge splurge of the feel-good, mind-enhancing protein BDNF (brain-derived neurotrophic factor) to boot.

TURN UP THE INTENSITY

Your heart will work really hard for short periods of time when sprinting (yellow), compared to at a steady level for a long period of time when jogging (orange). The lasting benefits for your heart are better after short bursts of exercise.

KEY

▬ Bursts of sprinting

▬ Steady jogging

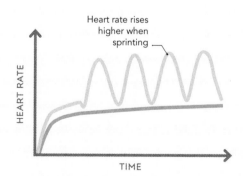

Heart rate rises higher when sprinting

HEART RATE

TIME

Does Exercise Make My Brain Fitter?

Exercise increases blood flow, delivering extra fuel to the brain. But getting your blood pumping delivers a host of other brain benefits, too.

Exercising to put your body under strain also makes the brain perform better. Today, we may run for the buzz, but for our ancestors, running was usually to escape imminent danger. Exertion drains the blood of glucose; deprived of its preferred fuel, the brain enters survival mode and prepares for the worst, suspecting mortal injury. First, brain cells generate a protective protein called BDNF (brain-derived neurotrophic factor). This softens the connections between brain cells, improving your ability to think, learn, and remember—which is essential when fleeing from danger.

New brain cells can even grow under the influence of BDNF—particularly in the memory hub of the hypothalamus—something that was thought impossible a few years ago.

Exercise makes the brain happy, too. Straining to squeeze that last ounce of power out of your legs when cycling up a steep hill isn't pleasant. With insufficient oxygen-filled blood flow to meet the maximum push, muscles become acidic and painful. Your brain's solution for the agony is endorphins: the body's homegrown morphine. Endorphins first reduce pain then deliver a rebound "high" as they continue to squirt through the blood after the pain subsides.

ONE HOUR OF HIIT
TRAINING PRODUCES MORE **ENDORPHINS THAN ONE** HOUR OF **AEROBIC EXERCISE**

It doesn't stop there, though; regular aerobic exercise, such as jogging or swimming, brings harmony to the brain's chemistry, and the resulting mood lift can be equivalent to taking antidepressant medication. Brain cells produce more of the messenger chemicals (neurotransmitters) GABA and glutamate—both of which are in short supply in people with severe depression and which play a major role in regulating mood.

What's the Best Exercise to Burn Calories?

Losing weight simply means burning more calories than you eat. The sums seem simple, but reality isn't always easy, especially when it comes to our efficient bodies.

The number of calories we burn varies according to our size, weight, gender, fitness, and muscle mass, so it can be very tricky to calculate exactly how many calories a person is using up during exercise. Calorie counts on fitness trackers and gym machines don't take these individual differences into account. They're all based on averages and are notoriously inaccurate so should be taken with a pinch of salt. Experienced distance runners, for example, typically burn

5–7 percent fewer calories than novice runners for the same distance and pace, because novice runners have yet to develop a smooth, efficient technique.

You may have heard that low-medium intensity exercise, such as jogging, is the best way to burn calories because you are working out in your "fat-burning zone" in which your body "chooses" to burn fat because, that way, it doesn't need to plunder the fast-acting glycogen stores

GO HARD OR GO HOME

If you walk two miles in an hour, you'll burn about 200 calories, with roughly 140 of them fueled by fat. Cycle moderately for that period, and you'll burn about 500 calories, with about 250 of them from fat.

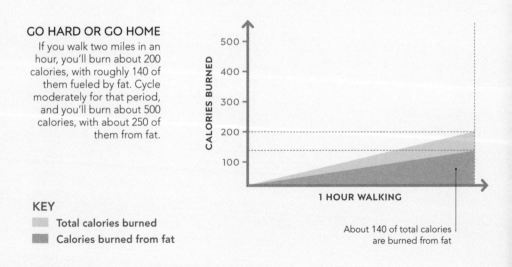

CALORIES BURNED

500
400
300
200
100

1 HOUR WALKING

About 140 of total calories are burned from fat

KEY

Total calories burned

Calories burned from fat

in the muscles. It's a nice idea, but sadly it's not true; the body eats into fat stores at roughly the same rate whether you're jogging or just walking briskly.

CALORIE COUNTERS
ON **FITNESS** TRACKERS ARE **INACCURATE** BY
UP TO **30**%

Things go a little better for fat burning when you exercise at full tilt—then you will be burning more calories overall, so more of those calories will be coming from your fat stores.

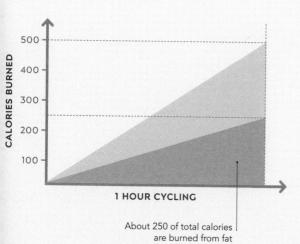

CALORIES BURNED

500
400
300
200
100

1 HOUR CYCLING

About 250 of total calories are burned from fat

WE'RE ALL ENDURANCE RUNNERS

We are the best long-distance runners on the planet, a fact that has helped us conquer the world. A deer will leave you in the dust if you chased after it, spear in hand, but there is a good chance you could outrun the sprightly hoofed animal in an ultra marathon.

Called persistence hunting, our hunter-gatherer ancestors were able to catch and kill faster and stronger animals simply by chasing them doggedly all day until their quarry collapsed with exhaustion, at which point they would close in to kill their prey. We've evolved to be the most efficient traveler of any other land animal. Your hips, shoulders, and limbs are perfectly balanced to swing effortlessly, propelling you forward with barely any effort. This economy of movement uses as little as possible of our stores of precious energy— and is precisely what makes losing weight by exercise alone such a long slog.

How Do I Trade My Belly Fat for a Six Pack?

The belief that you can target particular areas of the body to get rid of unwanted fat is an enduring myth that serves only to keep ab-blast gym classes in business.

The principle of "spot training" or "spot reduction" is, unfortunately, nonsense—belly fat (or indeed any areas of unwanted fat) can't be banished by repeated squats or abdominal crunches. Fat cannot turn into muscle; they are two very different, independent tissues. Fat is a bumpy, yellow tissue, made up of millions of cells called adipose cells, each containing a tiny droplet of fat. Muscles are long, protein-filled, electrified red fibers that shorten and thicken when they contract.

When you exercise, your body uses up fat reserves from all over the body—not necessarily from the area that's doing the work

ONE OF THE **BEST EXERCISES** TO BUILD **AB MUSCLES** ARE **CRUNCHES** ON AN **EXERCISE BALL**

To remove all doubt, a study at the University of Massachusetts saw a team of volunteers go through a 27-day training program of sit-ups, whereby each person crunched more than 5,000 times a day. Thanks to the extra exercise, their fat tissue reduced—each droplet of oil in the adipose cells shrinking slightly—but the shrinkage was equal right across their bodies.

Spot reduction exercise, if it is intensive enough, might seem to work at first because fat *is* lost in the target area, but you'll notice that fat is also lost all over the body.

So to return to your bothersome belly fat—if you undergo weeks of sweaty ab crunches, your abdominal muscles will indeed be more visible, but you might have got there even quicker with a different fitness regime.

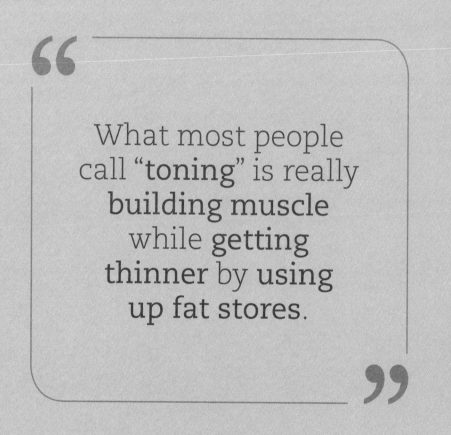

"

What most people call "**toning**" is really **building muscle** while **getting thinner** by using up fat stores.

"

What's the Best Way to Build Up Muscle?

You might think you're building muscle as you exercise, but the body doesn't start bulking those biceps until after you've put the weights away.

Almost all the muscles in the body are made up of two main types of fibers: the bulky, heavy-lifting type, known as "fast-twitch" fibers for their bulletlike contraction speed; and the slender, super-efficient, "slow-twitch" endurance fibers.

Fast-twitch fibers in your leg and arm muscles are the gas-guzzling supercars of the muscle world. Capable of immense strength and speed, they have limited staying power, due to their small fuel tank and feeble blood supply. They burn fuel faster than oxygen can get to them so can become quickly overwhelmed by the acid and chemical leftovers from the body's fuel-burning process.

If you want to build your brawn, push your muscles to their limit quickly by lifting weights and straining the muscles' fast-twitch fibers. Lifting weights inflicts dozens of microscopic tears in these fibers, which cause the aches and pains you feel afterward—the scientific jargon for that is DOMS (delayed onset muscle soreness). This soreness serves an important function: it's your body's way of persuading you to stop using your muscles until they

Muscle tear

BUILDING MUSCLE
When you rest after a workout, your muscle fibers absorb new cells and grow larger. Every time you train and rest, the process repeats itself.

MUSCLE FIBER
BEFORE EXERCISE

MUSCLE FIBER
AFTER EXERCISE

are fully recovered. When you rest, your body starts to repair the tears in the muscles. An army of baby muscle cells (called satellite cells) glide in to help repair the tears. The new cells are then fused into your muscles, making the repaired muscle a little bigger and stronger than before. Repairing and rebuilding can happen properly only when the muscle is left to rest, and that's why your muscle-building regime must always include rest days between workouts.

There's a spike of muscle-growth hormones in the afternoon, so it's best to plan your workouts for then to maximize the amount of muscle you build. Lowering your weights gracefully is more important than how you heave them up. Concentric muscle contraction occurs when you lift a dumbbell; whereas eccentric muscle contraction occurs when you slowly lower a dumbbell back down. Eccentric muscle contraction causes more microscopic tears than concentric, so you'll get stronger quicker if you lower weights slower than you lifted them.

Gone are the days when a water bottle and towel were the only gym essentials; today, a protein flask has become a workout must-have. However, most people get ample protein from a balanced diet. For all except top athletes and bodybuilders, consuming extra protein is usually unnecessary. It won't give your muscles a magical boost, and if you take in more than you need, that pricey protein simply disappears down the toilet bowl as urine. Unused protein is also converted into calories— around 130 calories for one scoop of a typical protein powder—so it can be an easy, but unwelcome way to put on weight.

700 THE TOTAL NUMBER OF MUSCLES IN YOUR BODY

Satellite cell helps repair and rebuild muscle

Satellite cells mature into muscle cells, fusing to the muscle to add bulk and strength

MUSCLE FIBER
DURING REST

REPAIRED
MUSCLE FIBER

How Do I Avoid "Hitting the Wall"?

Exercise should be one of life's great pleasures. Finding a balance between challenging your body to perform better and pushing too hard can be tricky.

Every one of your body's tissues and organs gets the energy it needs by burning glucose flowing in the blood. This supply is continuously replenished by energy stores in the liver and muscles, made up of another form of sugar, a starch called glycogen. You wouldn't go on a long car trip without a full tank and so neither should you embark on a long race without full fuel reserves. If you're exercising on empty, then you can expect to "hit the wall" quickly—legs suddenly go wobbly; you

feel light-headed, weak, and confused; and you might collapse. You're scraping the bottom of the barrel of your body's glycogen reserves. Body and brain grind to a halt as the fuel tank runs dry and blood sugar suddenly plunges.

THE **BLOOD** OF A
154 LB (70 KG)
PERSON CARRIES **JUST 4G**—ONE TEASPOON— OF **SUGAR**

BODY FUEL TANKS
When you are well fed, you have around 100g of sugar (as glycogen) in the the liver and 500g in the muscles. This is enough to fuel around four hours of steady exercise before blood sugar can no longer be topped up and you "hit the wall".

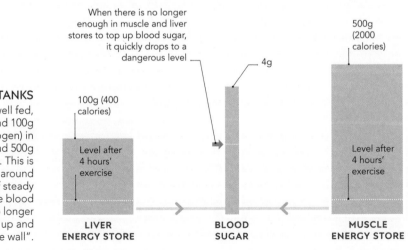

When there is no longer enough in muscle and liver stores to top up blood sugar, it quickly drops to a dangerous level

4g

100g (400 calories)

Level after 4 hours' exercise

LIVER ENERGY STORE

BLOOD SUGAR

500g (2000 calories)

Level after 4 hours' exercise

MUSCLE ENERGY STORE

"Hitting the wall" is potentially very dangerous, so it's important as soon as you feel any symptoms to stop, refuel, and rest. If you're going to be exercising for more than an hour and a half, take some easy-to-digest carbohydrate fuel with you—such as sugar-containing gels, drinks, or sweet snacks such as small blocks of chocolate or sweets—and eat something every 45 to 60 minutes. The snacks will replenish you so that you don't come close to hitting the wall.

As long as you're well nourished when you set out, you won't need to eat anything during the first 60–90 minutes of exercise.

WANT TO **AVOID THE WALL?**

1
SUPER-LOAD YOUR MUSCLES and lessen your intake of carbohydrates in the week leading up to a big race so that your muscles are "craving" to be filled.

2
EAT LOTS OF CARBOHYDRATES the day before the event to ensure your body's fuel tanks are full. Science shows that just one day of this "carb-loading" is enough to maximize the amount of starch your body will store.

3
GO FOR ISOTONIC DRINKS—they have a similar sugar level to blood and so are absorbed quickly, keeping "the wall" at bay for longer. Make sure you still drink plenty of plain water, though.

BURNING UP EXERCISE MYTHS

When you're gasping for breath on your spin bike, you may hear the gym instructor yell, "Take it to the burn!" to encourage you to burn fat faster. This burn, we are told, is a buildup of "lactic acid" and a sign that muscles are working at their limits. Not true. Lactic acid does not cause the pain; it's your friend—a product of the body's desperate attempt to calm the chemical inferno raging inside the muscles. The "burn" is actually caused by waste chemicals clogging up muscles being pushed to their limits, and it's perfectly normal to feel it when you exercise. It shows your muscles are doing their job to clear out the junk.

Also, when that instructor tells you to take deeper breaths in order to take in more oxygen, it's not true—you'll take in the same amount of oxygen as on a regular breath. The real reason you take deeper breaths is to get rid of all that carbon dioxide. However, the spinning class instructor yelling at you to "breathe harder to blow off your exhaust!" doesn't quite have the same motivating ring to it.

Is Socializing Good for Me?

It's natural to want to spend time with others—when socializing, the brain releases hormones that build bonds, and its neural networks are relaxed but sprightly.

Navigating the social norms of a large gathering requires a large, fast-working brain. We started to develop our oversized, socially aware brains about 2 million years ago, when we lost our fur and used the protein in our diet to build gray matter instead. This delivered an added bonus: our faces were more visible, revealing subtle facial movements and blushing. We could then more easily broadcast the richness of our emotions to the world, which helped us form bonds with one another and build successful, socially cooperative communities.

The brain pathways that ignite when we socialize are almost identical to the brain's "wandering mode" network. As the room hums with conversation, a crowd of areas across the brain co-operate so as to immerse us in the lives of others. "Listening" and "watching" regions are at work, as well as hard-thinking sections, without

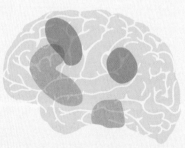

OUTER BRAIN

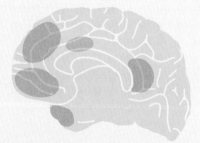

CROSS SECTION OF BRAIN

PARTY BRAIN

Your brain buzzes with activity in company: the amygdala sparks emotional awareness; the empathy network and mirror neurons (see right) help you identify with others; and the mentalizing network helps you understand social interaction.

KEY

- Amygdala
- **Mentalizing network**
- Empathy network
- **Mirror neuron network**

which we would blurt out the first thing on our minds. Also alight are the reward areas that make talking feel good. Our social-thinking pathways crackle as they anticipate others' thoughts, feelings, and actions, just like how we predict the path of a thrown ball.

This hubbub of gray-matter activity can make our health flourish. Meeting people and sharing good times releases a dual dose of the feel-good hormone

PEOPLE WHO DON'T SOCIALIZE
HAVE UP TO 60%
INCREASED RISK
OF DEVELOPING
PREDIABETES

dopamine as well as the attachment hormone oxytocin, helping you form bonds with your friends. Regular volleys of feel-good brain chemicals are often an antidote to anxiety, lowering stress hormone levels. Research shows that those who regularly interact with a circle of friends and family are happier and have better physical and mental health. Exercising empathy and caring, it seems, brings balance to emotions.

Conversely, a life of solitude can be unpleasant and even hurtful; the symptoms of rejection and isolation are so similar to physical pain that they can even be relieved with painkillers.

ARE YOU COPYING ME?

Spend a day with someone who has a strong regional accent and by the evening, you may find yourself speaking with a similar twang. We intuitively copy those around us, not to mock or out of a deep-seated insecurity, but because the brain is predisposed to make you mimic others.

If you see someone banging a drum, the same brain pathways fire as if you were actually doing the hitting. When you see someone in pain, the areas in your brain that register pain give you a mirror image of what you believe they are experiencing.

This is due to a pathway of brain cells called "mirror neurons." These seem to run alongside your normal pathways and reflect what you see in others. They're the source of your mimicry: you can learn to play the guitar by watching someone else; you'll automatically smile when others smile at you; and you'll unconsciously start to speak and act like those around you. This, of course, helps you blend in and become part of the group.

Why Am I Unluckier Than My Friends?

There is no Lady Luck, only your outlook on life's uncertainty. "Lucky" people tend to see events as opportunities rather than obstacles, and it seems that can make a big difference.

In one study, 400 volunteers were asked whether they considered themselves lucky or unlucky, and then they were given a truly tedious task: counting the number of photos in a newspaper. Self-confessed unlucky people took several minutes to count the 43 images, while the lucky cohort folded up the paper within just a few seconds.

Researchers had inserted an advertisement on the second page of the paper: "Stop counting—there are 43 photographs in this newspaper." Lucky people tended to spot the ad, whereas the luckless didn't register it. They also didn't spot the second large message halfway through the paper stating: "Stop counting, tell the experimenter you have seen this and win $250." The research concluded that those who considered themselves lucky people have a positive outlook and watch out for new possibilities.

A positive mindset is no cure-all and neither is cynicism the bedfellow of a happy life. However, if you are open to chance opportunities, avoid fretting about a fixed goal, and have positive expectations, you are much more likely to be able to transform "bad luck" into a string of lucky wins.

KEEP IT WIDE
"Lucky" people are more likely to be optimistic and open to new ideas; those who are "unlucky" tend to be more anxious, narrowing their mental focus and blinkering themselves to potential opportunities.

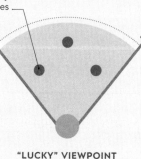

Wide focus; more likely to spot opportunities

"LUCKY" VIEWPOINT

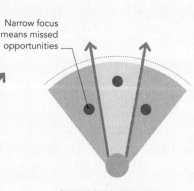

Narrow focus means missed opportunities

"UNLUCKY" VIEWPOINT

How Can I Be a Better Judge of Character?

More often than not, your instinct when meeting someone new will be to trust first and doubt second. Our innately trusting natures make spotting a liar difficult.

From the moment you emerge from the womb, you're wired to trust your parent. Trust is the cornerstone of civilization, and without it, society would never have advanced. Our innately trusting natures mean we can love, build friendships, and offer and receive care. Alas, they also make us rich pickings for con artists to take us for a ride.

Be under no illusion: you can't spot a liar. "Experts" may claim that they can spot when someone's lying by looking for a "tell," such as a touch of the nose or a facial twitch. However, decades of research show that even professional interrogators can't tell whether someone is telling the truth any better than those relying on chance alone. Lie detectors (known as polygraphs) are similarly hopeless because they detect fluctuations in heart rate so are able to detect only when someone is anxious—and people can be perfectly calm and still able to lie.

Interestingly, the more we pay attention to visual cues, the less able we are to gauge what is being said. Dishonest politicians can find that their untruths are more likely to be picked up in a radio interview rather than on TV.

95%
OF STUDENTS IN A SURVEY THOUGHT THEIR **ABILITY** TO **SPOT DISHONESTY** WAS **BETTER** THAN AVERAGE

WANT TO BE BETTER AT SPOTTING LIES?

1

CLOSE YOUR EYES and listen just to a person's voice. Your brain can judge someone better when not processing facial expressions.

2

LOOK OUT FOR SHORT SENTENCES and avoidance of words such as "I," "myself," or "personally"—both of which are common signs of lying.

3

LISTEN CAREFULLY to what you're being told, be alert for inconsistencies, and weigh up the logic of the story.

Why Are Some People So Stubborn in Their Views?

No matter what you say, some people can't or won't soften their stance on an issue. We all have a tendency to be pig-headed, and our brain's energy-saving circuitry is to blame.

We've all been exasperated by someone who wholeheartedly believes something idiotic and seems unable to see the error of their ways. Weighing up information about a topic, event, or person to form a reasoned, logical opinion isn't easy—it calls on sprawling networks of brain cells to do some intense neural work. Your brain loves energy-saving shortcuts, so it's far more efficient to strengthen an existing thought pathway—such as the idea that people drive worse on Sundays—than it is to put the effort into softening the existing opinion and forming a new one.

RESEARCHERS FOUND THAT UP TO

69% OF **MEDICAL STUDIES** ARE AFFECTED BY **CONFIRMATION BIAS**

We all, therefore, unwittingly cherry-pick events and remember whatever bolsters our existing belief. If, for example, you believe (wrongly) that violent crime increases when there's a full moon, you'll selectively remember all the news reports of crimes that happened on a full moon and in turn forget the full-moon days that were crime-free. Detectives can easily be caught in this trap, forming a hasty opinion on the perpetrator of a crime and then looking only for evidence that points toward that suspect.

These thought processes are called "confirmation bias"—and all your beliefs and opinions are colored by it. This is why you tend to give more weight to people who agree with you and easily cast aside contrary opinions.

Take a conscious step back and understand that psychology is working against both parties—science shows that being aware of confirmation bias and putting yourself in each other's shoes can help debaters see sense. Weigh up the logic of what each party is saying and compare hard facts. Interestingly, the most effective technique for overcoming fixed thinking is to try to argue from the other person's perspective. Perhaps then that dinner-table political debate can truly be put to rest—but don't bank on it.

Is Hugging Good for Us?

Science shows that human beings are born to cuddle.
Everybody needs physical touch to boost both
physiological and mental well-being.

Practically every land-based mammal goes in for embracing its own kind—it's a behavior that has been passed down through evolution. Not only does it have the physical benefit of keeping youngsters warm and safe from predators, but it's also an expression of trust and intimacy.

Studies show that touching helps keep the body's internal chemistry balanced. Seconds after an embrace begins, the pituitary gland in your brain releases a surge of the cuddle hormone, oxytocin, into your blood. Spreading rapidly through the body and brain, this hormone reduces activity in the analytical parts of your frontal lobes and instead heightens empathy, trust, and generosity. It also lowers cortisol in the blood, which reduces any feelings of fear and anxiety, as well as numbing pain.

Also, hugging and physical intimacy offers the opportunity for people to breathe in each other's pheromones, potentially amplifying sexual attraction (see pages 174–175). In the wider animal kingdom, pheromones speak of alarm and aggression, lay down territorial boundaries, accelerate parent-child bonding, as well as indicate fertility and sexual compatibility.

Infants who receive regular tactile stimulation (for example, physical play and hugs) form stronger bonds with their carers and tend to have better sleep patterns than little ones who rarely cuddle. Research indicates that people who often embrace others have a more robust immune system, lower blood pressure, and more resilient mental health than those who don't.

BECOME A **HEALTHY HUGGER**

1

MAKE IT REGULAR—people who hug more are happier and healthier. Across cultures, hugs tend to last three seconds. Some research says that embraces that last 20 seconds give a particularly nourishing dose of oxytocin.

2

PETS COUNT! Amazingly, research shows that similar health benefits can be enjoyed from stroking a pet.

3

GO EASY ON STRANGERS—all the benefits of hugging are reversed when we hug someone we don't know.

Why Am I So Nervous Around Someone I Fancy?

When your heart is pierced by Cupid's arrow, you're rocked by an inner whirlwind, causing a flood of hormones to rush into your body and brain.

Countless poems and songs have tried to capture the giddy, almost sickening thrill of romantic love. It usually starts with a meeting of eyes. The heart thumps wildly as pulses of the fight-or-flight hormone, adrenaline, pound through the blood. Pupils enlarge, hairs stand on end, cheeks flush, and palms become sweaty. You get "butterflies in your stomach" (see page 199).

Changes also happen to your brain: the mind becomes locked in emergency mode. The brain enters a heightened "watching" mode, and you might find you're unable to think clearly. Your once-smooth demeanor disappears, leaving you stammering clumsy, ill-judged sweet nothings to your crush.

Quelling this tsunami of stress responses and regaining the power of coherent speech is not easy; try a deep, slow breathing routine to persuade your brain that there's no imminent danger (see page 110).

Pupils dilate

Your sense of smell will be heightened, and you may detect the other person's pheromones

Ventromedial prefrontal cortex analyzes their dating potential

Your cheeks will flush, making your attraction clear to your crush

Increased heart rate

THE SIGNS OF ATTRACTION

When you are attracted to someone, your brain leaps into action at once, lighting up a telltale constellation of bodily changes.

"

The sensation of **attraction** is so **similar** to **fear** that watching **a scary movie** can be a **good first date**—the fear brought on by the movie will **amplify your feelings**.

"

Why Do I Find Certain People Attractive?

The science of attraction is a biological game. There are patterns to what most people find attractive, but ultimately, it really is all about sexual chemistry.

Across cultures, the masculine and feminine physical traits that most people find most attractive are remarkably similar. Desirable masculine qualities include broad shoulders and a muscular, V-shaped upper body; feminine attributes are a curvaceous figure, full lips, and soft facial features. In a primitive and unconscious way, these features give us clues about who will make a good mate and parent of future children.

It's hard to deny that some people hit the genetic jackpot, and these good-looking types top the dating "league table." A psychological theory called "the matching hypothesis" explains how all of us are placed in a desirability pecking order, with the most biologically attractive people at the top. Research shows that people find their match with someone who has a similar position in the league table—beautiful people tend to get together with beautiful people, and so on. This hierarchy sounds simplistic, but real-life romance really does generally follow these rules. However, see pages 178–179 for some overriding factors.

Hormones are key players in attraction. When you're physically intimate with someone, you breathe in their pheromones—odorless, airborne messaging chemicals emitted from their sweat glands, breath, saliva, and other bodily fluids—and your hormones respond. Although it is difficult to pin down precise human pheromone chemicals, their effects are powerful; for example, if someone inhales vapors from a partner's tears, their testosterone level drops, blunting sex drive and making them more able to offer care and comfort.

Primal chemistry has an important part to play in attraction, and smell is crucial—you'll find some people's scent more aromatic and heady than others. If you're turned on by somebody's smell, you're detecting pheromones that hint

15 MINUTES

OF **BREATHING** THE **MALE PHEROMONE** ANDROSTADIENONE MADE **HETEROSEXUAL WOMEN** MORE **AROUSED** AND **HAPPIER** that your DNA is compatible because you have different immune systems. This means that, were you to have children, they would likely have strong immune systems. Your unique immune profile is contained in a collection of proteins called the major histocompatibility complex (MHC). If a potential lover's smell is a bit of a turnoff, it probably means your immune systems are too similar (and perhaps you are related). Curiously, MHC molecules also influence same-sex attraction.

In some cases, it's wise to be wary of trusting the first whiff. For example, science shows us that women taking the oral contraceptive pill have a flipped pheromone love sensor and tend to be drawn to less genetically compatible mates. Also, scientists have yet to pin down specific pheromones, so be suspicious of companies selling pheromone-instilled aftershave or perfume—you're likely buying a placebo rather than guaranteeing yourself a good first date!

Brain's limbic system controls a host of emotional responses when you're attracted to someone

PRIMAL PHEROMONES

Scientists have identified a tiny organ the size of a sesame seed called the vomeronasal organ (VNO). It detects pheromones, and it's connected to parts of the brain, such as the amygdala and limbic system.

Amygdala in the brain controls fight-or-flight response

Vomeronasal organ is a bundle of tiny nerves nestled in the nasal cavity

Is Being in Love Good for My Health?

Falling in love brings waves of hormones into play, each with their own powerfully uplifting, but sometimes compromising, effects.

Scientists aren't known for being gooey-hearted, but the ones who have trained their critical eyes on romantic matters have deduced that there are three strings to Cupid's harp: lust (the sexual urges that you feel), attraction (so that you find a good mate), and attachment (so that you stay together in the long term).

Lust first appears when you see someone you fancy and is also stoked by strong feelings of attachment. Sex organs in both men and women release testosterone, revving up your sex drive.

Once you've established mutual attraction, your brain's reward centers become awash with a euphoric wave of dopamine. This hormone is associated with addiction (see page 210), and it motivates you to pursue the object of your desire, like a bee to a pollen-laden flower. The restless dopamine drive goes hand in hand with the "love chemical" phenylethylamine (or simply PEA). This is the brain's homemade amphetamine (a chemical similar to the narcotic "speed"), and it intensifies your excitement. Also, the energizing hormone cortisol creeps up, putting an extra spring in your step.

Contrary to what you might expect, levels of the positive hormone serotonin actually take a dip, which seems to help provide the single-minded focus to pursue your Romeo or Juliet. Loss of

WANT TO MANAGE YOUR LOVESTRUCK SYMPTOMS?

1
CUT YOURSELF SOME SLACK—the heady cocktail of hormones will give you single-minded focus on your love. Other parts of your life, such as your job, may take a back seat.

2
TAKE SOME TIME OUT and make sure you spend time with other people. The dopamine drive can lead to unhealthy focus; men are at highest risk of becoming obsessive.

3
LOOK AFTER YOUR HEALTH because lack of sleep and an off-kilter appetite can take a toll.

4
BE REALISTIC—the initial rush of emotions is intoxicating, but this "madly in love" phase inevitably passes, no matter how strong the relationship.

"APHRODISIAC" FOODS HAVE ZERO IMPACT ON **LIBIDO** – ALL HAVE BEEN SHOWN TO BE **EQUALLY INEFFECTIVE** IN MEN AND WOMEN

appetite and disrupted sleep are common, the culprits being all that dopamine and another energizing hormone called noradrenaline.

What emerges from lust and attraction is attachment. This is when a couple's internal chemistries knot them together and calm the blazing fire. The cuddle hormone oxytocin—which is also released powerfully after sex—builds affection and bonding, reinforcing the loving feelings we have for our partner. Together with another hormone called vasopressin, it brings a sense of calm out of the brew of passion. Lust and attraction remain active within the relationship but are tempered by these calming agents.

Perhaps alarmingly, the electro-chemical soup in the mind of someone smitten by love has similarities to the brain of a person with obsessive-compulsive disorder (OCD). So although it's normal for a lover to be very preoccupied with their partner, it's worth noting that, when it comes to your brain, a romantic crush is only a stone's throw away from an out-of-control obsession—and this is why

being newly in love can feel so disconcerting, even threatening.

Generally speaking, the chemical boost you get from this assortment of hormones is good for you in that it lifts your mood and improves your motivation in other facets of your life, too. Falling in love can be overwhelming at first, but luckily, the hormonal storm does subside—peace will return.

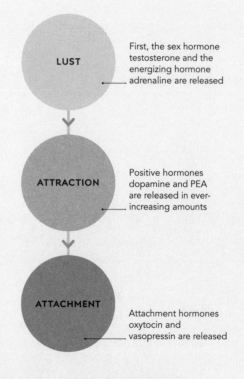

First, the sex hormone testosterone and the energizing hormone adrenaline are released

Positive hormones dopamine and PEA are released in ever-increasing amounts

Attachment hormones oxytocin and vasopressin are released

THE INITIAL COCKTAIL OF LOVE
Each aspect of being in love drives its own unique cocktail of hormones with a range of powerful effects on the body and mind.

What's Most Attractive in a Long-Term Partner?

The things we look for when we're choosing a life partner, whether consciously or unconsciously, often depend on our own status, sex, and sexuality.

A lasting romantic relationship has many strands, and sexual attraction is generally the first to show up. Science tells us that almost-symmetrical faces are what sets our hearts aflutter. Our biological urges may regard this symmetry as a very crude marker of good health and genes.

Biological beauty is important, but a degree of social currency is also very attractive to some. People who seemingly "cheat" the matching

hypothesis system (see pages 174–175) by gaining wealth, status, and power may zoom up the league table. Overweight, older tycoons might end up marrying someone much younger and beautiful. In terms of physical attractiveness alone, these matchups make little sense: none of the obvious evolutionary qualities mark out the tycoon as a healthy partner-in-the-making. Instead, security and influence compensate for any biological

LOOK FOR A PARTNER with similar interests and attitudes to social issues, money, politics, and other important facets of life.

UNDERSTAND the matching hypothesis—it's natural to be attracted to someone higher up the league table but it's not a guaranteed happiness.

CHERISH INTIMACY because loving, sexual contact early on is a feature of happy long-term relationships.

NURTURE YOUR LOVE
Every partnership has its trials and tribulations, but surveys tell us there are a few key components that will make the relationship stand the test of time.

"weaknesses." It appears that, when it comes to status, love can truly be blind.

Sexuality plays a part in attachment. Heterosexual women look for men with markers of high testosterone: mainly physical brawn (giving him the ability to intimidate others and protect the family) but also high cheekbones, a chiseled jawline, and a strong brow. For heterosexual men, part of a woman's allure is her ability to bear children: wide hips, large breasts, and soft features mean lots of estrogen. The pitter-patter of tiny feet may be years away from a first date, but the heterosexual sex drive has been honed to see the bigger picture.

Studies show that both straight and gay men place a higher premium on looks than social standing when seeking a long-term partner, whereas straight women tend to be influenced by a man's status. Gay women, on the other hand, tend not to be influenced by either and instead seek out honesty over all other traits.

Every union needs compatibility in order to go the distance—lust isn't enough to last. Rom-com fans might think that opposites attract, but this belongs firmly in fiction. Psychological research, online dating, and social media data prove that birds of a feather flock together, so your friends and partners are likely to share your attitudes on politics, religion, and morality.

53% OF **MEN** AND **43% OF WOMEN** IN ONE STUDY LISTED **THEIR SPOUSE** AS THEIR **BEST FRIEND**

NURTURE YOUR FRIENDSHIP by spending time together and pursuing shared interests to keep the attachment secure.

IT'S A CHOICE: make a conscious decision to commit to carry on loving another person, even when the initial thrill passes.

KEEP TALKING, because lovers who frequently share their feelings and worries, without fear of judgment, are more likely to stick together.

HAVE SEX OFTEN— one study showed that having sex weekly rather than monthly led to a happiness jump equivalent to earning an extra $50,000 a year.

Why Do I Get PMS and Period Pains?

The short—and rather shameful—answer is that scientists don't know enough about a process that half of the people on the planet experience every month for half of their lives.

Medical research has historically focused primarily on men, and most scientists (also mainly men) have simply ignored the "complication" of a woman's monthly cycle. This ignorance is universal: surveys show that globally, more than half of all people say they aren't properly taught why periods happen and what goes on in the body when they do.

WANT TO EASE **MONTHLY MISERY?**

1

GET PLENTY OF EXERCISE and eat a varied diet to lift your mood and buffer against irritability.

2

TAKE VITAMIN B6 AND CALCIUM supplements, both of which help the body counteract the worst symptoms.

3

TAKE A HOT SHOWER OR BATH to stimulate blood flow to the uterus, helping cramping muscles relax.

4

ASK YOUR DOCTOR about new treatments: for example, research shows that Viagra, used to treat male erectile dysfunction, may help ease period pain.

Human females are unusual; most other animals, apart from apes, don't have periods. Nobody knows quite why we are different—as with other animals, periods may be a way to wash out the womb and ward off infection, or it may be that the pregnancy-ready human womb lining is simply too thick to be reabsorbed into the body.

A yo-yoing mood, abdominal pain, acne, and tiredness in the week or so before a period is known as premenstrual syndrome (PMS). The syndrome is the butt of many a joke, and women are often reluctant to talk openly about symptoms. At this time, levels of sex hormones progesterone and estrogen plunge, causing a slump in mood, while simultaneously wreaking havoc on the balance of fluids in the body, causing bloating and fatigue.

During a period, abdominal pain is common. The muscles lining the uterus contract powerfully to expel the contents. This constricts tiny arteries to stem blood flow but also inflames nerves, causing cramping and pain.

> Unbelievably, **serious scientists** have publicly insisted that PMS is **"all in the mind"** of the **75% of women** who say they experience monthly mood swings.

Why Do My Periods Sync Up with Others'?

The idea that women who live together have periods together is older than history books, but science has shown that there is no invisible force that unites women in this way.

In the early 1970s, scientists believed that pheromones—odorless vapors that send messages between animals—were the reason women's menstrual cycles aligned over time.

However, research has now made it clear that, contrary to popular belief, period syncing simply does not happen any more often than by chance alone. The average menstrual cycle lasts 29 days, although there is huge variation between women, and cycles can range from 15 to 45 days. Intervals between periods also vary month to month, so two or more women will invariably have some months when they are in sync and others where they're not. It's the times when your periods fall on the same days that tend to stick in your memory—it's as simple and unmystical as that.

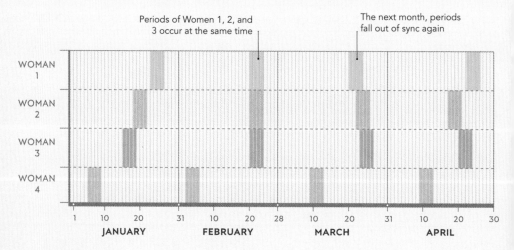

Periods of Women 1, 2, and 3 occur at the same time

The next month, periods fall out of sync again

JUST COINCIDENCE
The calendar shows how the monthly cycles of four women vary from month to month and naturally fall in and out of sync over a four-month period.

How Can I Manage Menopause?

Bearing children in old age is risky, so flicking the fertility switch to "off" is for your and society's benefit. The key might be not to manage menopause but to celebrate it.

Female humans are among the very few animals whose biological fertility clock expires long before they do. Around the age of 50, a woman's periods become irregular and gradually stop. This is menopause, and as our hormones effect this change, so can some uncomfortable symptoms start.

Hot flashes are the most well-known symptom. When the supply of female sex hormones drops after the last good egg has been released, the body's thermostat suddenly becomes very temperamental. Normal temperatures can feel uncomfortably warm, and a slight increase in ambient temperature can set off a bout of feverish sweating. Other symptoms include headaches, anxiety, sadness, dry skin and hair, and a loss of sexual desire.

Interestingly, studies show that women who welcome menopause as a new phase in their life are significantly less likely to report severe symptoms. Symptoms also vary in different societies: in cultures where a woman's youthful looks and fertility are prized, physical side effects seem to be multiplied. In Japan, most women don't report hot flashes but instead a "chilliness." And in cultures where older females are respected, symptoms seem to cause much less mental anguish.

It's far too simplistic to conclude that menopause symptoms are down to the prevailing attitudes of society—your body is undergoing its greatest upheaval since puberty. But resisting shame and positively embracing the change can boost your chances of a flash-free menopause.

WANT A **MELLOW MENOPAUSE?**

1
AVOID OVERHEATING—at night, keep the bedroom cool and wear loose clothing (see page 43).

2
TAKE CARE OF YOURSELF by eating healthily, exercising regularly, and getting some sunlight. Try relaxation techniques, such as mindfulness meditation.

3
SEE YOUR DOCTOR—some women undergo HRT (hormone replacement therapy) to replenish the lost supply; it can significantly relieve severe symptoms.

Is There Such a Thing As a Midlife Crisis?

There's no age limit on making rash decisions—we can lose the plot at any point. But middle age, when the pressures of life peak, is often a time to take stock and reflect.

When you think about a midlife crisis, chances are you are thinking of a 40-something man who has splashed wads of cash on a flashy car or motorcycle that can be heard half a mile away. In Western countries, about a quarter of 40+ adults claim in surveys that they have had a midlife crisis.

The idea originally came from a psychologist's theory that geniuses such as Mozart suffered a creative block in their mid-30s. American pop culture later attached the concept to impulsive middle-aged men.

In reality, there is no spike in irresponsible behavior in the 40s and 50s. We make good and bad decisions throughout life. That said, it is undeniable that middle age can be a challenging time, when life satisfaction reaches a gloomy low. Perhaps the slump is because this is often a time of maximum stress and responsibility in careers and family life. Most psychologists agree that our 40s and 50s are a time for taking stock of life, when we realize that we may not accomplish all our hopes and dreams. It may simply be that a bit of reflective gloominess is in our biology, because scientists have noticed that other primates go through a similar phase in their mid years.

Take heart, though—in older age, when responsibilities may be fewer, our contentment grows again steadily.

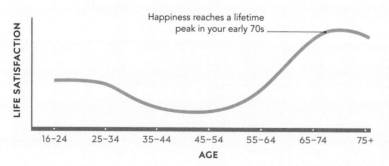

Happiness reaches a lifetime peak in your early 70s

LIFE SATISFACTION

16–24   25–34   35–44   45–54   55–64   65–74   75+

AGE

IT GETS BETTER
Surveys show that in Western countries, life satisfaction reaches a low between the ages of 44–46, rising steadily again until you reach old age.

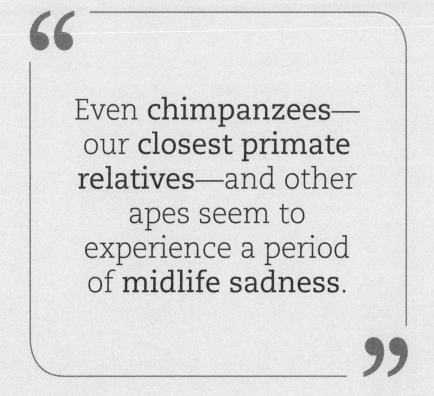

> Even **chimpanzees**— our **closest primate relatives**—and other apes seem to experience a period of **midlife sadness**.

Can I Blame My Bad Mood on Hunger?

If you get tetchy before dinner, science offers you a cop-out for your tantrums. You really can blame your body chemistry for making you "hangry."

In evolutionary terms, being "hangry" makes sense. An animal that gets aggressive when hungry will be a better hunter. But in today's world, it's less helpful when you're stuck in traffic and late for dinner. This reaction is the same one that tempts you to skip lunch and power through the post-lunch slump on adrenaline only.

When the stomach is empty, the body produces the substance neuropeptide Y. The happy hormone serotonin dips under the influence of this messaging chemical, making us single-minded, focused, and irritable. In addition, the brain's limbic system, our center of emotions, becomes volatile when

THE WORD "HANGRY" WAS OFFICIALLY ADDED TO THE MERRIAM-WEBSTER DICTIONARY IN 2018

blood sugar drops. And to cap it all, hunger hormones from the stomach power down the self-control circuits in our frontal lobes, making us impulsive.

They say, "Never go to bed angry"; it would be similarly wise to not make big decisions or settle a quarrel on an empty stomach—being hangry really is a thing.

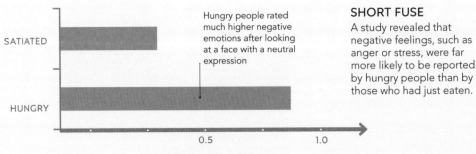

Hungry people rated much higher negative emotions after looking at a face with a neutral expression

SATIATED

HUNGRY

0.5   1.0

LEVEL OF NEGATIVE FEELINGS

SHORT FUSE
A study revealed that negative feelings, such as anger or stress, were far more likely to be reported by hungry people than by those who had just eaten.

Is Eating a Large Meal in the Evening Bad for Me?

The science isn't as clear-cut as some evangelical nutrition gurus would have you believe, but nonetheless, eating large and late won't enhance your health.

It is often claimed that eating late will make you put on weight. Strictly speaking, this isn't true—it's the calories you eat and burn over the entire day that determine weight management. That said, late eaters are more likely to be overweight than those who eat earlier, but this is because they also tend to lead less active lives and choose more fatty, high-calorie foods more often.

The later it gets, the weaker your self-control and the more impulsive you are. This can mean evening meals are larger than they need to be or that your impatience leads you to opt for a high-calorie "quick fix."

Try planning dinners ahead of time to help avoid making impromptu, hunger-driven decisions. We're creatures of habit—especially where food is involved—so look out for patterns of evening overindulgence (such as eating and drinking alcohol while cooking). Alcohol not only contains calories but also makes us hungrier by dialing up the brain's appetite centers. Regularly eating large meals at nighttime does not seem to be good for overall health.

During the dark hours, your body clock is winding down all systems into standby mode—including your intestines. Eating very late can disturb the body clock, leading to disrupted sleep. This in turn pushes up blood pressure and, ultimately, can damage your blood vessels and heart.

However, a small meal or snack late at night is not harmful and may actually be helpful for elderly people, those recovering from injuries, or athletes looking to improve their strength and general fitness.

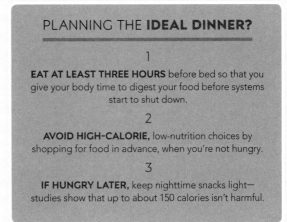

PLANNING THE **IDEAL DINNER?**

1

EAT AT LEAST THREE HOURS before bed so that you give your body time to digest your food before systems start to shut down.

2

AVOID HIGH-CALORIE, low-nutrition choices by shopping for food in advance, when you're not hungry.

3

IF HUNGRY LATER, keep nighttime snacks light—studies show that up to about 150 calories isn't harmful.

Why Is Everyone Putting On More Weight?

Every year, levels of obesity are rising globally. It's not fair to say we've devolved into greedy monsters with no self-control—it's the foods sold to us that are the problem.

Since 1975, the obesity rate has tripled globally; in children, it has increased sevenfold. If we carry on as we are, by 2030, one-third of the world will be overweight. If you're an adult living in the US, UK, Mexico, Canada, or Hungary, and you aren't overweight, then you're in the minority. So why are we all getting bigger?

It's not because of a famine in mental fortitude and self-control.

IF YOU'RE OBESE, YOUR LIFE EXPECTANCY MAY BE REDUCED BY 12 YEARS

We humans are food-driven animals who have found ourselves in a world where tasty, fat-filled, sugary food is available on every street corner, supermarket aisle, and menu. Plus, this kind of food is sold to us at a price that makes it a compelling choice for those of us who are short of both time and money.

Compounding this, our bodies don't make it easy for us; not only do our stomachs release hungry hormones whenever they're empty—regardless of whether we need the food—but we're all biologically programmed to throw rational thought out the window when we eat foods high in the unholy trinity of sugar, fat, and salt (see pages 92–93). Our bodies seek out this type of food and we love it in the short term but pay for it with our health in the long run. Biologically speaking, we're getting a raw deal.

After stopping smoking, shedding some pounds if you are overweight is the single best thing you can do for your health. Being obese not only shrinks your life span but reduces the number of healthy years you'll enjoy.

Staying active is critical for good all-around health, but exercise can claw back only some of your lost years if excess body fat isn't lost. Sadly for many, weight loss is easier to pontificate about than it is to achieve. Only fairly recently has science turned to the issue of just why so many of us find it nigh-on impossible to shift excess weight. One thing is sure—answers are urgently needed to reverse the crisis.

CAN I HAVE SOME MORE?

Fast-food outlets and food manufacturers in the US have progressively increased portion sizes over the past 70 years. The average fast-food meal offering now contains up to four times more calories than its 1950s precursor.

KEY

🔵 Portion sizes in 1950

⬤ Portion sizes in 2020

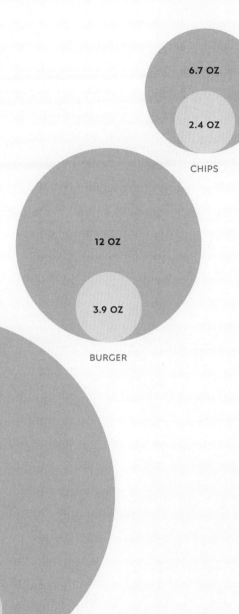

6.7 OZ

2.4 OZ

CHIPS

12 OZ

3.9 OZ

BURGER

42 OZ

7 OZ

COLA

Should I Use BMI to Aim for My Ideal Body Weight?

BMI is a reasonable guide to a healthy weight, but to get a more accurate and personal picture of the ideal weight for you, you'll need to dig deeper.

We know that fat tissue is an essential part of our body makeup and serves several important roles, but how do you know when you've got too much? Ask a health professional or personal trainer, and they will likely point you to BMI (body mass index)—a number score that measures your weight while taking into account your height.

Your BMI will tell you whether you are significantly overweight or underweight. It's also a useful marker for governments to "guesstimate" how much of their population is carrying

too much fat or is undernourished. While you *can* use BMI to roughly calculate whether you are over- or underweight, beware—when it comes to using your score to figure out how much of the excess weight you are carrying is fat, BMI is decidedly flaky. It doesn't take account of muscle, which is heavier than fat, and neither does it adjust for height properly—if you're tall, your BMI will be overinflated; if you're shorter than average, your BMI will be unduly low. You can easily have a BMI outside the

HELPFUL GUIDE

BMI is calculated as your weight in pounds divided by the square of your height in inches multiplied by 703. Doctors usually say that for an average adult, a BMI between 18.5 and 24.9 indicates a healthy proportion of body fat.

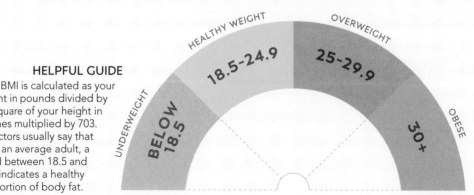

HEALTHY WEIGHT

OVERWEIGHT

18.5-24.9

25-29.9

UNDERWEIGHT

BELOW 18.5

30+

OBESE

recommended range (see below) and be in peak fitness.

The best way to find out how much fat you're carrying under your skin and wrapped around your organs (the latter being the most harmful to health because it disrupts the body's insulin control) is to have a body scan. However, since few will be able to access a scanner, "smart scales" are a relatively inexpensive alternative,

A 6 FT (1.8 M) **OLYMPIC ATHLETE** WHO WEIGHS **212 LB** (96 KG) WILL HAVE A **BMI OF 28**, MAKING HIM "OVERWEIGHT"

which give reasonably reliable results. When you place your hands and feet on the panels, the scales use small electrical currents to estimate the proportions of fat, water, and muscle in your body.

A newer, more accurate formula to calculate body fat than BMI is relative fat mass (RFM), which is a ratio taken from your height and waist measurements. It's easy to do—all you need is a tape measure—and there are plenty of online calculators to crunch the numbers for you.

BMI IS BELGIAN— WHO KNEW?

Like a hallowed scripture, few people question the BMI scale and its weight categories. However, in reality, the formula is a 200-year-old math hack, originally based on the sizes and weights of sedentary Belgians—and badly in need of an update.

In the 1800s, a statistics-loving Belgian astronomer, Adolphe Quetelet, wanted a neat way to figure out how many Belgian people were obese—and it turned into a bit of an obsession for him. In an era without calculators or computers, he devised a simple formula to find what he was after: a rough and ready "fatness" score that accounted for people's height.

Life insurance companies soon cottoned on to the idea that they could turn the data into tables showing the "average weight"— and charge higher premiums for anyone who was "overweight" or "obese." A hundred years later, Quetelet's formula was rebranded as "body mass index" by Ancel Keys—the famous American nutrition scientist.

I Eat Well, So Why Can't I Manage My Weight?

We're notoriously poor at judging how much (or how little) we are eating. The chances are that your estimation of "normal" is off the mark.

Everybody knows someone who eats bowls of ice cream and seemingly never puts on an ounce. Quite why many of us seem to gain weight just by nibbling the odd chocolate pick-me-up has long been a mystery. Might the slender-framed among us have a faster metabolism, greater willpower, or just be born with skinny genes (letting them fit into their skinny jeans)?

It seems much of it is down to human error. We're terrible at judging how much we've eaten, most of us significantly underestimating the number of calories we eat in a given day—even when we keep a food diary. Sugary drinks, milky coffees, that midmorning treat, and the evening glass of wine are easily (and conveniently) forgotten, but they all add up. (Interestingly, studies show that people living with anorexia consistently overestimate the calories in their food.)

Neither are we given bodies that put us on a level playing field. You have your own unique basal metabolic rate—the amount of energy your body burns just to keep you alive. Generally, the younger and more muscular you are, the more calories you burn. Two identically proportioned people will have different metabolic rates, although it rarely varies by more than about 200 calories per day (equal to a glass of full-fat milk). Nevertheless, this may be

WANT TO **SHED THE POUNDS?**

1

EAT SMALLER PORTIONS—by simply putting less on your plate, you have less chance of overeating.

2

REGULAR EXERCISE is critical for good all-around health and short bursts of high-intensity workouts are typically the most efficient for burning surplus fat.

3

KEEP A FOOD DIARY and don't let anything slip under the radar. Studies have found that keeping a photographic record of food eaten delivers better weight-loss results than a conventional diary.

4

MODERATE ALCOHOL INTAKE—not only are alcoholic drinks high in calories and low in nutrition, but they also impair judgment, making your already-dodgy internal calorie counter even more of a liability.

enough to explain why your slim friend can get away with eating an extra dessert each day.

Achieving this balance between food intake and your personal metabolic rate can be a constant challenge. On average, everyone gains about 1 lb (0.5 kg) every year, but we can't blame a falling metabolism; our weight creeps up mostly because we exercise less as we get older.

We know that obesity is too much of that good thing called fat, but too little body fat can be just as harmful. When body fat drops below 5 percent of your total weight (around 25 percent is average), your tank is running desperately low. The body will turn down its central heating and save energy by switching off your fertility and sex drive. Hair, nails, and bones stop growing. In extreme cases of malnutrition, your body may even resort to digesting its own organs, such as the liver, simply to stay functioning— effectively burning the house's furniture just to keep warm.

Body fat in itself is not the enemy— quite the contrary. Fat keeps you warm (see page 46), stores lots of vitamins, and provides a truly vast stockpile of fuel to keep you going come rain or shine.

PEOPLE WHO KEEP A **FOOD DIARY** TYPICALLY UNDERESTIMATE THEIR FOOD INTAKE BY

33%

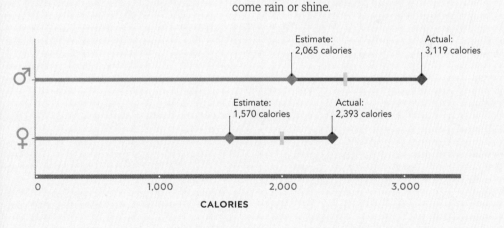

ESTIMATED VS. ACTUAL CALORIES
In a study, people's reports of their daily calorie intake was compared to what they actually ate. Almost everyone underestimated—and men were slightly more inaccurate than women.

KEY
▬ Self-reported consumption
▬ Actual consumption
▬ Recommended daily amount (RDA) of calories

Are Fats Good or Bad for Me Now?

In the last century, no foods have suffered more fluctuating fortunes than fat. Recent science points to evidence that most fats are more sinned against than sinful.

Since the mid-1950s, fats have been blamed for obesity and many other health woes. Much of this fat blaming has turned out to be baseless and motivated by marketing, not science (see page 95). Low-fat diets in one form or another dip in and out of fashion. They can be effective in the short term, although they may throw up other health issues (see below).

There are two main different types of food fats, and many fats and oils contain both. Saturated fats are easy to spot because they're solid

1 GRAM OF FAT
CONTAINS **9 CALORIES**; 1 GRAM OF SUGAR CONTAINS JUST **4 CALORIES**

at room temperature—think cheese or the rind on a pork chop. They come mainly from animals but are also found in coconut and palm oils. Eating too much can lead to high levels of harmful cholesterol. Floating through the bloodstream, cholesterol soaks into the

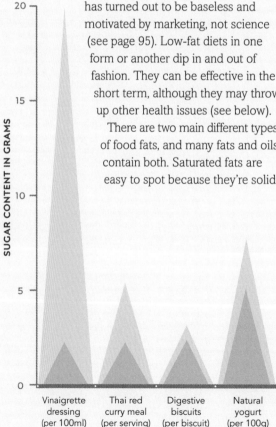

KEY
■ Regular version
▧ Low-fat version

LOW FAT, HIGH SUGAR
If you compare the sugar content of some processed foods with low-fat versions, the result can be a shock. Reduced fat means less taste, so many manufacturers compensate by adding sugar—and plenty of it.

SUGAR CONTENT IN GRAMS

20

15

10

5

0

Vinaigrette dressing (per 100ml)

Thai red curry meal (per serving)

Digestive biscuits (per biscuit)

Natural yogurt (per 100g)

GOOD FAT SOURCES

- Plant oils, such as olive, sunflower, or rapeseed oil
- Some nuts, particularly almonds, Brazil nuts, and peanuts
- Avocados
- Seeds, such as sesame and sunflower
- Oily fish, such as salmon, trout, and sardines

walls of arteries, eventually clogging them—much like pouring too much bacon fat down the sink will block your drain. Conversely, unsaturated fats, which are usually liquid oils at room temperature and are found mainly in fish and plant-based foods, do not cause a buildup in the same way—they may even help keep arteries clear and are linked to good heart health.

Like coals on a fire, fats provide long-term energy and also cause the "gut brain" to quickly lower hunger levels. Fats are also essential to provide the building blocks for nerve sheaths and a range of hormones as well as the outer coating of every cell in the body.

Strictly speaking, fats don't even make you fat! They do, however, make food taste great, so it's tempting to eat more than you need. Low-fat versions of common foods can be a bad choice, because the extra sugar and salt added to offset the blandness can cause weight gain.

THE HERO THAT BECAME A VILLAIN

The heart attack is a disease of modern times. Once an obscure medical emergency, by 1960, one in three American men were dying of heart disease, and everybody blamed saturated fats.

The hunt was on for a heart-healthy alternative to butter, so scientists set to work. This led to the creation of an ingredient that could rightly be considered a poison—partially hydrogenated oils, also called trans fats. Creative chemists devised a way to turn liquid vegetable oils into semisolid, spreadable fats, which looked like butter (after yellow colorings were added). This alchemy was accomplished by bubbling hydrogen gas through vats of heated vegetable oil mixed with nickel.

However, in the 1990s, studies proved these trans fats to be deadly; fat-processing machinery in the liver mutates them into bad cholesterol, accelerating the buildup of fatty deposits in arteries faster than any slab of butter.

Most manufacturers now don't use them, but it's always worth double-checking labels for these Frankenstein fats—and avoiding them at all costs.

Is My Weight Genetically Programmed?

Most of us are born with the chips stacked against us having a super-lean physique—our genetic code makes us adept at converting excess food energy into fat.

Your genes decide whether you will be tall or short, a born marathon runner, or predisposed to high blood pressure and heart attacks. And at least 50 of your genes determine how good you are at accumulating a padding of fat. For example, if you have an abnormal version of a gene called MMP2, your body can create body fat quicker than most. Around a third of women have this fat-building gene. Such people are blessed when faced with famine but cursed in our world of cheap, fast food.

Another gene, FTO, sets the gauge on how much pleasure you get from eating by determining how much of the hormone dopamine is released when you eat. People who carry a particular version of this gene are 20–30 percent more likely to be obese and will be on average about 3 lb (1.5 kg) heavier than

ABOUT **90**%
OF US HAVE **GENES** THAT
MAKE THE **BODY BETTER**
AT CONVERTING EXCESS
FUEL INTO FAT

noncarriers. You are not powerless, though—research shows that regular exercise can negate the effects of a belly-building, faulty FTO.

Where you store the extra weight, however, is largely out of your control. We are each genetically programmed to stow our rainy-day blubber in different ways. Those who store fat subcutaneously (under the skin) are described as pear-shaped—their fat sits mainly on the hips, thighs, and arms. Apple-shaped people accumulate fat around their abdominal organs (known as visceral fat), giving them a round belly. Belly fat stifles the organs' ability to keep sugar levels balanced and blood-vessel pipework running cleanly, meaning that "apples" are more at risk than "pears" of type 2 diabetes and heart disease.

There's no quick fix for this; liposuction and surgery can't target visceral fat. The good news, though, is that better sleep, reduced stress, and regular aerobic exercise are all very effective in freeing organs from their fatty coverings.

" In **countries** with the **highest obesity** rates, **most** of the **population** carries a **gene** that **delivers** extra pleasure from eating food. "

Can Gut Microbes Help Me Manage My Weight?

Microbes in the gut feed on the food we eat, and in addition to providing a host of health-boosting services, they can help prevent obesity.

Microbes live all over your body, and trillions of them live in your gut. Although they are responsible for the malodorous gas we all love to hate, gut microbes are to be encouraged—they help the body extract nutrients from food, produce essential vitamins, calm an overactive immune system, reduce inflammation, and even bolster your defenses against less helpful, disease-causing organisms.

Researchers have recently discovered that gut microbes also play a big part in how quickly you gain weight. They found that people who are obese or who eat lots of highly processed food carry more kinds of superpowered, food-digesting bacteria. These microbes seem to help the body suck more energy than normal from each slice of cake, making it easier for you to gain weight.

Whether these fat-promoting bugs cause obesity or they proliferate as a result of being overweight or eating refined foods is an unanswered question; it is likely that both are partly

UNREFINED FOODS

HEALTHY GUT MICROBES
Candida
Bacteroidetes
Firmicutes

FAT-PROMOTING MICROBES
Blautia obeum
Lachnospiraceae dorea
Ruminococcus

PROCESSED FOODS

IMPROVE YOUR GUT HABITAT
Research has shown that a diet of highly processed foods is associated with gut microbes that make you prone to gain weight. Eating mainly unrefined, plant-based foods means fewer obesity-associated bacteria.

KEY
▬ Healthy weight
▬ Overweight

true. What we do know, though, is that by feeding your gut more vegetables, fruits, nuts, and seeds, these obesity-associated bugs will dwindle, helping your weight management efforts.

Keeping your gut microbes happy boosts your general health and makes weight management easier. Eating plenty of fiber is especially important—it's the microbes' favorite food. When bacteria in the colon ferment fiber to extract energy, a by-product of the process helps you absorb beneficial minerals, including calcium and iron. The bugs also secrete vitamin K, which helps the blood clot.

Probiotic foods, which contain live "helpful" bacteria, can add to a depleted microbe army, if the dosage is high enough. However, if you are well, probiotics are of little use—taking them is like trying to grow corn in a rainforest!

Take antibiotics only when you have to; they don't discriminate between friendly or enemy bacteria, so may wipe out the dutiful denizens of your gut.

PROBIOTIC PROS

- *Lactobacillus rhamnosus* may reduce allergies and helps weight loss.
- *Lactococcus lactis* may help protect against and treat diarrhea.
- *Lactobacillus plantarum* may reduce symptoms of irritable bowel syndrome.
- *Bifidobacterium bifidum* may help lower cholesterol.

BRAINS IN YOUR BELLY?

The entirety of the gut—from gullet to anus—is coated with a brainlike mesh of nerves that functions much like the gray matter in our skull. This second "brain" orchestrates the digestive process, and, incredibly, it could do the job even if it were completely detached from our brain. Our belly really does have a mind of its own.

The gut brain also responds to our emotions, becoming upset when we are distressed. Terror—such as we might feel just before an exam, an interview. or public speaking—can trigger an emergency bowel evacuation. This is the gut's effort to off-load excess weight before we have to flee. Hormones and nervous impulses that are released when we are anxious, stressed, or depressed instruct the gut brain to slow down or stop completely. It's no surprise then that mental illness often goes hand in glove with a range of abdominal and digestive problems, and there is a well-established link between a stress-filled life and irritable bowel syndrome.

Which Is the Best Weight-Loss Diet?

There is no perfect way to shed excess fat, although there are plenty of very bad ways. The trick is to sort the good science from the bad—and to be patient.

The equation is simple: if you put less fuel into your body than it needs, it will burn its excess fat. But the reality is that many of us find this incredibly difficult—and there are a number of methods and theories telling you how best to do it. Many diets are based on restricting certain food groups; for instance, gram-for-gram, fat carries more energy than protein, so a low-fat diet will reduce how many calories you take in. But precisely because fats are so calorie-dense, they can keep you full for longer, helping with weight loss.

Cutting out carbohydrates works because foods high in protein are more

10% OF THE **WEIGHT YOU** LOSE ON A CRASH DIET IS **MUSCLE, NOT FAT**

filling than starchy foods—consider how much easier it is to scoff a medium portion of carb-rich chips than it is to polish off two chicken breast fillets (a high-protein food with almost no carbohydrates), even though both contain the same amount of energy.

Rapid weight-loss programs are problematic; mental health often takes a hit, and risks of obsessive thinking are high. Also, quick weight loss means that muscle, as well as fat, is lost. Also people tend to regain weight just as quickly, leading to a vicious cycle of yo-yo dieting. As boring as it sounds, research proves that the best and most lasting results are achieved when weight is lost gradually through progressive lifestyle changes (reducing food intake and moving more).

BEWARE OF **"DIET-SPEAK"**

- **"Clean/raw food"**: Something that harks back to a "purer" past might sound appealing, but if you ate only raw foods, you'd struggle to stay fully nourished.
- **"Natural"**: Chemicals or additives are not all bad—everything that we eat is technically a "chemical," and additives can help keep food fresh.
- **"Science"**: Diets such as the "detox" or "acid-alkali" diet may claim to be backed up by science, but it's pure make-believe.

DIET	THE DETAILS	THE SCIENCE	DOES IT WORK?
CALORIE COUNTING	Staying within a set daily limit of calories—no food groups specifically restricted.	If the body takes in fewer calories than it expends, it burns stored fat.	Yes, although studies show that most dieters regain some or all weight.
INTERMITTENT FASTING	Very limited or zero calories on some days; eating normally on others.	Reduces calorie intake dramatically without shocking your body, possibly accelerating the burning of fat.	Yes, although some studies show mixed results. We don't yet fully understand the positive or negative effects of this diet.
KETOGENIC	Low carb, high in fat and protein.	Starving the body of its favorite energy (glucose) forces it to break down fats and protein instead.	Yes, although side effects include low energy, dizziness, headaches, vitamin deficiencies, and gallstones.
PALEO	Lots of meat, fruits, vegetables, and "fruit oils." No dairy or processed foods.	Based on the false idea that our hunter-gatherer ancestors ate a healthy diet. In truth, limited diets meant they were diseased and malnourished.	Yes, although high fat levels can cause arteries to fur up, and lack of variety may cause vitamin and mineral deficiencies.
ATKINS	Minimizes the intake of carbohydrates, particularly refined flours and sugars.	Cutting out carbohydrates was thought to force the body to burn more fat. Theory has been disproved.	Yes, although diet is hard to stick to. Also, high-fat meat-heavy diet is not ideal for overall health.
VERY LOW CALORIE	Drastically slashes food intake by replacing meals with liquids such as celery water or cabbage soup.	Often marketed by celebrities, these diets will leave you dangerously short of vital nutrients.	Yes, although it causes rapid destruction of fat and muscle alike, putting your body into a dangerous "starvation" mode.
DETOX	Focuses on juices and superfoods to cleanse toxins that accumulate in the body.	The kidneys and liver are highly capable of eliminating harmful substances, so these "cleanses" do nothing.	No. You may lose weight if you are eating less overall, but your body isn't being "detoxed."
ACID-ALKALI	Choosing foods that offset the body's natural acid-alkali balance.	The acidity of your fluids is tightly controlled by your body so this is unnecessary.	No.

WHAT'S ON THE MENU?

Many "branded" diets do deliver weight loss but at a cost of a range of side effects—some of them potentially serious. It's always wise to consult a medical professional before embarking on a weight-loss regime, because they can offer support and advice.

What's So Good About the Mediterranean Diet?

Scientists agree it's the closest thing to the best diet, although to get the full benefit, you don't just have to eat like the Italians and Greeks—you have to live like them, too!

A healthy mind, body, and long life is wedded to a good, balanced diet, and the two cannot be easily teased apart. When medical professionals distill nutritional science, research points toward what is loosely termed the "Mediterranean diet" as one of the healthiest of the bunch.

However, "Mediterranean" in this context doesn't mean a banquet of French cheeses, creamy carbonaras, and chocolate fondants, all washed down with copious bottles of red. This food regime is actually based on traditional Greek and Italian cuisine, harking back to a time when food was fresh, seasonal, and simply prepared and cooked— and the modern processed food industry wasn't even a twinkle in humanity's eye.

WANT TO LIVE **LIKE A MEDITERRANEAN?**

1

EAT A WIDE VARIETY of fruits and vegetables, with moderate amounts of protein, mainly fish.

2

CONSUME PLENTY OF NUTS, seeds, and legumes such as beans and lentils.

3

USE GOOD-QUALITY OLIVE OIL as the main culinary fat; eat only limited amounts of milk and animal fat.

4

AVOID PROCESSED FOODS and limit sweets and sugary desserts to occasional treats.

5

BE PHYSICALLY ACTIVE, outdoors if possible, as part of your daily routine.

6

GET AMPLE, UNDISTURBED SLEEP, topped up with an afternoon siesta.

AIM TO EAT TWO PORTIONS OF **FISH PER WEEK**, ONE OF WHICH SHOULD BE **OILY**, SUCH AS **SALMON** OR **SARDINES**

“

It's **not just about food**; it's the complete package of the **Mediterranean lifestyle** that **scientists recommend**.

”

Will Being Vegan Make Me Healthier?

Given that eating meat helped humans survive the rat race of evolution, is plant-only living healthy? The answer is yes, but you need to understand what you are eating.

Vegans were once seen as oddballs in the developed world, but a triple threat of ethical, environmental, and health concerns have led to a mushrooming of no-meat diets. In some countries where meat-eating was the norm, there has been a five- or sixfold growth in veganism in just a few years.

Even though it's clear that eating meat significantly contributes to the storm cloud of climate change, research shows that for most of us, the main reason to make the switch is not to save the planet—it's the promise of better health that gives us the nudge.

Generally speaking, the fewer animals and the more plants we eat, the happier our internal biology is. Plant-based diets have been linked to lower rates of obesity and longer, healthier lives. The more meat we eat – particularly red and processed meat— the higher our chances of heart disease, bowel cancer, and type 2 diabetes. However, simply cutting out meat, fish, and dairy without swapping

NUTRIENT	Vitamin B12 is vital to repair DNA and enable cells to burn energy.	Iron is used by blood cells to absorb oxygen from the air in the lungs.
	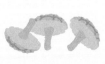	
PLANT-BASED SOURCES	Found very rarely in dried shiitake mushrooms, some algae and seaweeds, as well as nutritional yeast.	Found in nuts and pulses, leafy greens, and whole grain bread.

WHAT DO I NEED?

If you're moving to meat-free living, it's important to know where to get these nutrients from. In some instances, such as for vitamin B12, you might need to take a supplement, or choose fortified foods (those that have had the nutrient safely added).

them for sensible alternatives is a recipe for miserable malnourishment. Many life-essential nutrients are easy to come by in an omnivorous diet but all too easy to miss when living solely off flora. To enjoy a healthy transition to meat-free living, you'll need to keep a handle on crucial nutrients you could be missing out on.

Your body struggles to absorb some nutrients, such as iron or calcium, from plants because they are tightly wrapped in molecular parcels that even your powerful gut can't digest. Eating foods rich in vitamin C helps release iron from its leafy shackles, but in general, vegans need to be aware of their intake of iron and the other nutrients below—especially pregnant women, children, and those who are ill or recuperating. Taking vitamin supplements can be a good option for some (see pages 40–41).

IT STARTED WITH A PIG

Millions of people abstain from animal products for cultural and religious reasons and have done so for millennia. In the West, modern veganism began with a 13-year-old English boy named Donald Watson. In 1923, while staying at his uncle's farm, he was so horrified at seeing a pig being slaughtered that he vowed never to eat meat or fish again. Later, he expanded this to include dairy products, and then the wearing of leather, wool, or silk. He even used a fork rather than a spade when gardening so that he wouldn't accidentally slice any earthworms in two. In the 1940s, he founded the Vegan Society to campaign for his beliefs. Today, the society claims that there are 600,000 vegans in the UK alone.

Calcium promotes strong teeth and bones, keeps nerves firing and the heart beating.

Can be obtained from calcium-set tofu, fortified soy, rice, oat drinks, dried fruit, and leafy vegetables such as broccoli and cabbage.

Iodine is essential for the production of thyroid hormones, which regulate your metabolism.

Plentiful in seaweed, as well as in iodized salt (salt with added iodine).

Omega-3 fatty acids keep arteries clear, reducing the risk of heart disease.

Found in flaxseed and rapeseed oils, soy-based foods, and walnuts.

Why Is Nutrition Advice Always Changing?

When it comes to nutrition, scientific advice has a habit of flip-flopping—not only because of food-industry dollars but because the science itself is so slippery.

Given how much is written and said about healthy eating—the countless magazines, podcasts, books, websites, TV shows, and even university degrees—you'd think that scientists know a lot about what a healthy diet looks like. You'd be wrong.

Most of the healthy-eating advice spooned out by the multibillion-dollar healthy-eating industry is about as stable as a half-baked soufflé. Even dedicated scientists admit that we have only morsels of truly solid scientific fact when it comes to what foods will help us live longer. Health advice is always flip-flopping because nutritional science is so imprecise.

In an ideal world, researchers would collect a huge group of volunteers and randomly split them into smaller groups and then give each group a diet to follow. They would keep tabs on everybody for many decades, recording any notable differences in health between the sets of people. Simple though it sounds in principle, such research would be impossible and prohibitively expensive. It's hard enough

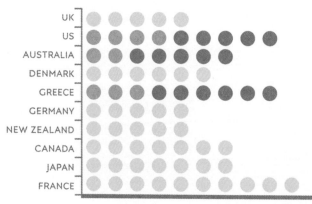

RECOMMENDED PORTIONS PER DAY

IS IT 5 A DAY OR 10?

There has never been a study that shows that eating a set amount of fruits or vegetables each day makes you live longer. Each country looks at the available research on healthy intakes and advises accordingly.

KEY

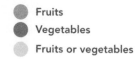

Fruits

Vegetables

Fruits or vegetables

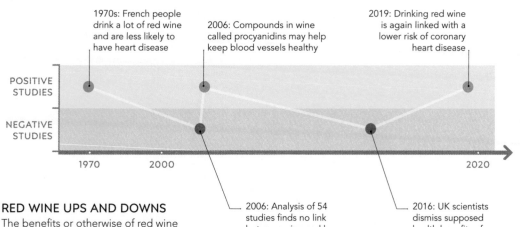

1970s: French people drink a lot of red wine and are less likely to have heart disease

2006: Compounds in wine called procyanidins may help keep blood vessels healthy

2019: Drinking red wine is again linked with a lower risk of coronary heart disease

POSITIVE STUDIES

NEGATIVE STUDIES

1970   2000   2020

RED WINE UPS AND DOWNS

The benefits or otherwise of red wine is a popular research topic—resulting in a timeline of fluctuating fortunes as conflicting studies are published.

2006: Analysis of 54 studies finds no link between wine and lower risk of heart disease

2016: UK scientists dismiss supposed health benefits of red wine

for one person to stick with a diet for six months—only 50 percent of dieters manage it—let alone for a group of hundreds to stay with a dietary regime for the 10 or 20 or more years needed to spot concrete health differences. Just imagine being told you had to eat a boiled egg every day for the next 20 years if you don't like eggs!

Most nutrition science, therefore, is based on surveys or food diaries, the results of which can be sliced and diced in many different ways. This can account for the seemingly yo-yoing advice. For years, studies seemed to prove that a glass of red wine or two every day was a healthy virtue (see above), leading to fewer heart attacks. However, more research showed such moderate drinkers are also likely to be wealthier, healthier, and lead a life filled

with sensible habits—which could account for their better heart health.

What we know for certain about healthy eating is that we should eat enough food so as not to be malnourished—but not too much, or else the excesses are turned into fat and we become overweight.

It has also been proven beyond all doubt that there are certain nutrients we must eat to stay healthy: these are essential substances that the body needs but cannot generate itself—vitamins, minerals, some fats, as well as certain proteins that contain amino-acid building blocks needed for the body to repair and grow. Lack any one of these, and your body will over time start to sputter and break. But after that basic nutritional know-how, almost everything else is just educated guesswork.

Why Do I Get Scared by Music or Sounds in Movies?

Whether it's the roar of a T. rex or the low, two-note tune of a shark on the hunt, smart filmmakers know that some sounds will always activate our built-in danger systems.

A creaking door, a howling wind—then suddenly, a bloodcurdling scream and discordant crash of piano keys reverberate through the building. It isn't just you—everyone else in the theater has just jumped out of their seat as well. Some things are plain scary, whether the danger is real or not.

Being jumpy at spooky sounds is in our DNA. Outside our control, the ever-alert amygdala hears something it interprets as dangerous and puts the emotional system on edge. Our adrenaline-fueled fight-or-flight reflex makes our heart race, blood pressure climb, hairs stand on end, and pupils dilate. (We know that if a person's amygdala is damaged or removed, they do not feel fear.)

When we are tense, a sudden noise makes us jump. We involuntarily blink (to protect our eyes) and our shoulder and neck muscles rapidly contract (to protect the back of the head). We share these shock and fear reactions with most of the animal kingdom.

Screams of panic or terror have a primal panic-inducing power. They are remarkably similar in all animals, tending to be loud and shrill, with a high pitch (or frequency) that wobbles up and down. We find some other sounds scary or shocking because they mimic a scream, such as the screeching of car brakes, the wailing of an emergency siren—or the jarring, staccato violin chords in a horror movie.

It's not just loud noises that set us off. Edge-of-your-seat creaky floorboards are similarly frightening because they seem to unlock the intuition of our fretful forebears: if we weren't vigilant to the quiet crack of a twig indicating an approaching predator, we would have become tiger food. Similarly, a howling wind puts us on edge because it masks these subtle noises, making us deaf to an approaching beast. (This is why many animals in the wild stop moving when a strong wind is blowing.)

WE ARE **HARDWIRED** TO **JUMP** AT A SUDDEN **NOISE** OF **80 DECIBELS** OR **LOUDER—** SUCH AS AN ALARM CLOCK

Movie composers have perfected the art of playing on all our scared-animal predispositions. We tend to be afraid of loud, low frequency roars and booms because in the natural world, there's a good chance it was made by something big and dangerous. Slow, low-pitched tones evoke tension and worry so a low, throbbing baseline sound played over a tense scene amplifies the sense of unease. Some movies even play ultra-low frequency "infrasound" notes (less than 20 hertz) that are imperceptible to us yet may still accelerate our fight-or-flight response.

Many of us enjoy horror movies because in the safety of the theater, that primal rush of adrenaline is felt as excitement rather than terror. We allow ourselves to enjoy the highly energizing effects of the fear response, while keeping a sense of control.

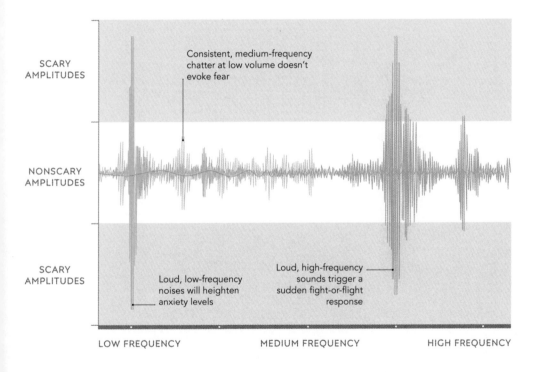

SCARY AMPLITUDES

Consistent, medium-frequency chatter at low volume doesn't evoke fear

NONSCARY AMPLITUDES

SCARY AMPLITUDES

Loud, low-frequency noises will heighten anxiety levels

Loud, high-frequency sounds trigger a sudden fight-or-flight response

LOW FREQUENCY   MEDIUM FREQUENCY   HIGH FREQUENCY

FREAKY FREQUENCIES

In common with most animals, humans tend to be afraid of sudden and loud noises at either extreme of the audible frequency range, such as the roar of a wild animal or a human cry.

KEY

— Human scream
— Normal conversation
— Lion's roar

Why Is Social Media So Addictive?

Social media notifications cash in on the chemical currency of pleasure: dopamine. When you're looking for "likes," you're single-mindedly focused on the next hormone hit.

Slot machines are said to be the "crack cocaine" of gambling—the emotional reward when you finally get a win after many tries is often far greater than the financial one. The same "one-more-go" compulsion is behind why some people obsess over social media updates, can't stop checking emails, or are forever playing video games. These compulsions are all driven by that familiar brain chemical, dopamine.

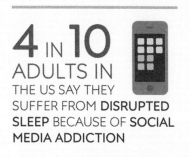

4 IN 10 ADULTS IN THE US SAY THEY SUFFER FROM **DISRUPTED SLEEP** BECAUSE OF **SOCIAL MEDIA ADDICTION**

Dopamine, released by the nucleus accumbens in the brain, is the "well done" of the sports coach that makes you glow with pride and the motivation for us to take action. In fact, animals that have no dopamine in their bodies don't even have the impetus to get up and eat.

Social media "likes" or "follows" may not be food, sex, or money, but someone else's admiration can still offer you an ego-boosting dopamine lift. Like the random payouts of the slots, there's no way of predicting when someone out there will reward you with their approval, so you'll impulsively keep checking in, hoping to see those likes stack up. Perhaps one day, you think, you might even win the dopamine jackpot—a thumbs-up from a celebrity or social media "influencer!"

WANT TO CURB THAT **ADDICTION?**

1

USE A SCREEN-TIME CHECKER that tells you how long you spend on apps—the shock can be a powerful motivator to cut down.

2

REMOVE ANY APP that you check impulsively. Try living without it for 30 days and see if you really want it back.

3

GET A NONDIGITAL HOBBY—studies show that more creative hobbies deliver more dopamine pleasure than digital ones.

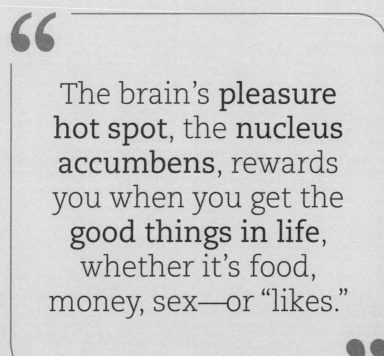

" The brain's **pleasure hot spot**, the **nucleus accumbens**, rewards you when you get the **good things in life**, whether it's food, money, sex—or "likes." "

How Can I Swap My Bad Habits for Better Ones?

Our habits are formed away from the control of the brain's conscious, decision-making frontal lobes—and their deep neural connections can't be severed overnight.

Deep in the brain, habits form in the "habit hub" in the basal ganglia—the same place that muscle memory forms (pages 130–131). Each time you perform a certain action, your brain releases the "well done" hormone dopamine. Over months or years of repetition, the neural connections between the habit hub and the reward centers strengthen, and for better or worse, the habit sticks.

A habit becomes a problem—or an addiction, if you will—when it causes us harm or we feel that we no longer have control over it or we need to do it in increasing amounts just to feel normal. Anything that delivers a particularly powerful dopamine boost has the potential to become your main source of pleasure. Drugs such as alcohol or nicotine ensnare people so well because they chemically deliver an unnaturally large dopamine release—up to 10 times the amount a "natural" reward does. The reward system is quickly hijacked, replacing the natural flow of dopamine so that we soon need the drug just to feel "normal" levels of pleasure.

The genes that determine our dopamine circuitry play a large part in how quickly we can become hooked on a habit, but our environment may

HOW HABITS WORK

All habits have a basic flow: you feel an urge to do something, you do it, it feels good, so you get the urge to do it again. If you have a snack most afternoons, soon a glance at the clock will trigger (or cue) your cravings.

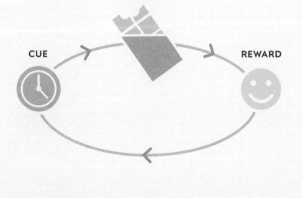

ROUTINE

CUE

REWARD

be equally important. We know that good connections with others and a sense of purpose and belonging makes dependency far less likely.

You may have heard that it takes 21 days to break a habit—alas, this is a piece of armchair-psychology nonsense from the 1960s. For daily habits such as drinking a glass of water after breakfast to doing 15 minutes of exercise a day, it takes an average of 66 days to stick—but others can take as few as 18 or as many as 254 days. How much the habit breaks your norm, your motivation to change, the satisfaction you feel, the complexity of the habit, as well as your individual personality, all have a bearing.

WANT TO LEARN
HEALTHIER HABITS?

1
AVOID NEGATIVE TRIGGERS, such as walking past a favorite bar. Instead, facilitate new triggers; for instance, put running shoes in plain view to prompt you to put them on and do some pleasurable exercise.

2
BREAK OR MAKE THE BEHAVIOR by simply doing the new habit as much as you can. Each time you do, you're strengthening the new neural connections in your brain, embedding the new routine.

3
NURTURE THE REWARD—if you take time to savor and appreciate the mood-lifting buzz of a new habit such as exercise, this can help a new fitness routine stick.

WHY IS SMOKING SO ADDICTIVE?

Nicotine—the highly addictive drug in tobacco—exerts powerful dopamine-pumping powers. Within seven seconds of you inhaling tobacco smoke, nicotine has bound to microscopic "nicotinic" receptors on brain cells, making the reward pathway fire feel-good pulses of dopamine. Although the taste is horrible, a few smokes over several days makes the brain produce even more nicotine receptors. We then must inhale ever-more nicotine to get the same pick-me-up effect—and cravings start when we try to starve these extra nicotine receptors. Smoking doesn't ease anxiety but merely quells the uncomfortable withdrawal symptoms generated by those needy receptors.

Around a third of people seem to produce more nicotinic receptors than others, making it extra hard for them to kick the habit. A lucky one in five people have a version of a pleasure-sensing "mu-opioid" brain receptor that seems to make ditching the cancer sticks a relative breeze for them.

NIGHT

As the sun kisses the horizon good night, so we hunker down for darkness. Twilight soothes the body after the day's demands, opening the door to calm. In this time for storytelling around the campfire, emotions are felt and shared effortlessly, and intimacy becomes easy. Eventually, slumber welcomes us with open arms and as we drift off; body and brain drink in the pure refreshment that only sleep can bring.

Is My Phone Ruining My Sex Life?

Everyone seems to agree that sex isn't as popular as it used to be. Are we too busy, too tired—or just too much in thrall to our smartphones to make time for intimacy?

Survey after survey confirms we are having less sex than ever before. Since the 1990s, couples have been increasingly finding the bedroom an intimacy-parched zone. Rates of teenage pregnancy have plummeted across developed nations in line with this apparent lack of libido: the fraction of people making love at least once a week fell from 45 percent in 2000 to 36 percent in 2016 in the US—and this "sex drought" has many people worried.

Smart devices are a prime suspect as a cause; their popularity has soared while romance's has sunk. Given that every new technology gets blamed for social ills, it may be a coincidence. Although there's no rock-solid scientific evidence that logging on is turning us off, evidence does point to those digital distractions subduing our sex life.

Intimacy is a bubble that's easily burst. Like a dog that learns to bark at the sound of the doorbell, so your brain quickly learns that a digital "ping" is your virtual doorway to the outside world. The sound is tethered in your memories to friends unseen and emails

IN ONE SURVEY, **30**% OF PEOPLE **ADMITTED** THEY HAD **ANSWERED** THEIR **PHONE DURING SEX**

unanswered. As if someone really were knocking on the door, fight-or-flight responses are tickled, instantly flicking your brain into its highly vigilant "watching" brain network (see page 70). This mindset is the antithesis of love and openness because it narrows your focus. Studies have shown that even the presence of a phone, regardless of whether it is used, can make people less empathetic toward those they are with.

A smart device, even in airplane mode, can similarly sabotage the state of mind needed for love—and lust— to blossom. When you're planning a romantic evening, it may be prudent to leave the phone in the fridge when you go to take out the wine.

"When a **phone**—even if it is **turned off**—is on a table **near us**, our **face-to-face** conversations become **less caring** and lack **empathy** and **intimacy**."

Is There a Best Time to Have Sex?

Hormones take the reins of our sex drive, but culture, habits, and the routines of life mean that we can't always heed their clarion call—we have sex when we can.

In the natural world, few species appear to have sex for pleasure—we are in an exclusive club that includes dolphins and other primates.

Testosterone is a chemical cattle prod for sexual desire in both sexes, although it's significantly lower in women; for them, estrogen plays a bigger role in sexual desire.

Testosterone surges for everyone in the mornings, priming the body for sex. After orgasm, a cocktail of hormones imbue a relaxed, loved-up state, so sex in the morning could be a stress-busting, blood pressure–lowering start to the day. Also, the chances of conception are highest before 7:30 a.m., when sperm numbers and their swimming abilities are at their daily peak. If you need to be lively first thing, then beware: an almighty surge of the sleep-inducing prolactin after sex—particularly in men—means the urge to roll over and start snoring can be irresistible.

Your personal biological clock also has a say. Night owls are better primed for late-night loving, while morning types favor morning amour. Research shows that the couples who are happiest with their relationship often have body clocks that are synchronized to each other's sexual urges. Hormones are, of course, only one facet of sex drive—real life superimposes itself on

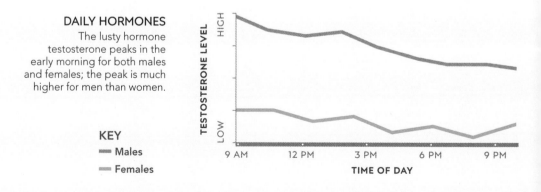

DAILY HORMONES
The lusty hormone testosterone peaks in the early morning for both males and females; the peak is much higher for men than women.

KEY
▬ Males
▬ Females

TESTOSTERONE LEVEL — HIGH / LOW

9 AM   12 PM   3 PM   6 PM   9 PM

TIME OF DAY

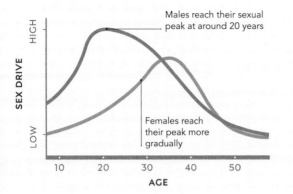

Males reach their sexual peak at around 20 years

Females reach their peak more gradually

SEX DRIVE · HIGH · LOW

AGE · 10 · 20 · 30 · 40 · 50

LIFETIME LIBIDO

On average, the male libido peaks at an earlier age than the female libido and reaches a higher level. Male and female desire is roughly equal in their 30s and again in their mid- to late 40s.

KEY

━ **Males**

━ **Females**

this chemical impulse. Couples tend to have sex when opportunity strikes—intercourse rates are highest at night, when both parties are conveniently lying in bed together.

11:30 PM IS THE TIME WHEN COUPLES ARE MOST LIKELY TO HAVE SEX

As well as the daily hormones, the roller coaster of sex hormones over months and years holds huge sway over your libido. For women, sexual desire rises and falls broadly in line with fertility. It rises in the first half of the monthly cycle, which is the prime time for baby-making—even if sperm arrive before an egg is launched, they can happily tread water for five or so days. After egg release, the passion-killer hormone progesterone dampens lust in the second half of the cycle.

Men also have their own, simpler

rhythm of sexual desire. For example, after seven days of abstinence, sex-seeking testosterone surges, before returning to a steady level.

Science shows that even seasons affect procreative sex; sperm are healthiest and fittest in the springtime and most feeble in summer.

New parents often find they're at the mercy of libido-blunting chemical changes. Sex hormones dip in new mothers, and testosterone similarly slumps by 26 to 34 percent for new fathers—even their testicles shrink! Research shows that this temporary halt on testosterone helps men be better, more attentive fathers. Remarkably, the brains of new parents rewire, retuning the dopamine-driven reward system to be more motivated toward childcare rather than sex.

There's no "best time" to have sex—but for a male/female couple in their 20–30s, on a spring morning in the first half of her cycle, a week after they last had sex, the odds are that having sex will be at the top of their "to-do" list.

Why Do We Yawn, and Why Are Yawns Contagious?

The curiously contagious yawn and its function are mysteries that have had researchers stumped. There are clues that yawning might be a leftover habit from our earliest times.

Yawning reveals more about you than you might think. Tiredness and boredom are the obvious triggers for an arms-outstretched, wide-mouthed yawn, but nervousness and worry are also causes—and why you might see an athlete yawning just before a big race. Even sexual arousal can set off yawns—so don't be offended in a moment of intimacy!

IN ONE STUDY, **82%** OF **UNDER 25-YEAR-OLDS CONTAGIOUSLY YAWNED**, COMPARED TO ONLY 41% OF OVER-50S

So what does yawning do for us? This is a puzzle that researchers never tire of trying to solve. Some myths have been dispelled: low oxygen levels don't trigger a yawn, and yawning doesn't increase oxygen in the blood. Neither is it a way of cooling the brain when it's hot—in fact, breathing through the nose cools us more efficiently than a mouth breath.

What we do know is that we yawn most when we're feeling sluggish—at night, early in the morning, or when we're bored. A neat idea might be that it's your body's way of keeping you lively when your mind is drifting, but science has shown that this isn't the case—we're no more energized after yawning, and the electrical firing in the brain remains unchanged.

Perhaps there's a more primal reason. For much of the animal kingdom, showing off your teeth signals a "back off" message or warning. So although our teeth are puny, it's possible that yawning is a legacy from our animal ancestors and a way of showing the weapons we're packing when we're at our most vulnerable—tired or foggy-headed.

Why, then, are yawns contagious? We are empathic by nature: the areas of the brain that light up when you "catch" a yawn are the same ones that come alive when you care for and connect with others. Family members catch yawns more than strangers do—even dogs can catch yawns from their owners! Interestingly, children don't tend to catch them until age five—presumably because they haven't yet developed mature empathy circuitry.

" Studies show that **yawning** helps close-knit groups of social animals, such as the chimpanzee, to **synchronize** their **body clocks**. "

Do Sleeping Pills Help or Hinder?

Your body clock releases a range of sleep-inducing chemicals that helps you put head to pillow. Medication tinkers with this process so comes at a cost.

Any medicine or substance that hastens sleep—be it sleeping tablets or alcohol—actually hampers good sleep. Sleeping aids make you drowsy either by chemically tickling the sleep-inducing part of the brain called the VLPO or muffling the stay-awake impulses from the brain's RAS region. Drugs (and alcohol, see right) do send you to sleep, but medicated slumber is not the same as the natural kind. In fact, any chemical that makes you sleepier or more awake (including caffeine) cripples the normal rhythm of sleep.

Like alcohol, sleeping pills tend to pull the plug on REM sleep while also railroading you into medium-depth sleep and bouncing you out of the most restorative deep sleep, thus starving you of sleep's full healing potential. Medications are, however, useful in the short term. When combined with good sleep hygiene, they can help guide a broken sleep pattern back into a healthy routine.

Melatonin supplements are often trumpeted as a "natural" remedy for sleep issues, but this is based on a

ABOUT **33**%
OF **AMERICAN ADULTS** HAVE TRIED A **SLEEP DRUG** OR **SUPPLEMENT**

fallacy; melatonin isn't the hormone that makes you sleepy—it's actually adenosine that's responsible for the creeping tiredness that makes you want to drop off.

As the body clock senses the fading light, your body releases melatonin in the hours running up to bedtime. This signals winding-down time, rather like the ringing of an end-of-the-day school bell. Taking melatonin right before bed isn't useful at all—it's like sounding that bell in the middle of the day—all the students will assume it is a mistake. In the same way, a melatonin supplement taken when your body isn't tired won't speed your journey into slumberland—your body will know it's a false alarm and ignore it.

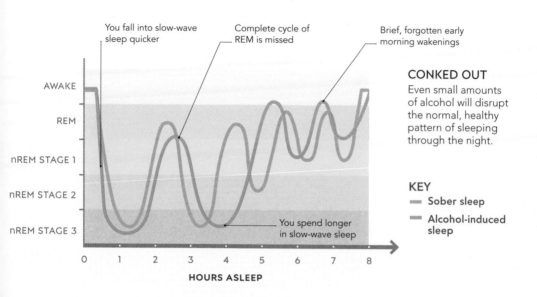

You fall into slow-wave sleep quicker

Complete cycle of REM is missed

Brief, forgotten early morning wakenings

CONKED OUT
Even small amounts of alcohol will disrupt the normal, healthy pattern of sleeping through the night.

AWAKE

REM

nREM STAGE 1

nREM STAGE 2

nREM STAGE 3

You spend longer in slow-wave sleep

KEY
— Sober sleep
— Alcohol-induced sleep

0   1   2   3   4   5   6   7   8

HOURS ASLEEP

Will a Nightcap Help Me Sleep Better?

On a chilly night, a hot toddy can seem the perfect way to glide you into the Sandman's soothing embrace. But however tempting, a fiery nightcap will always backfire.

Alcohol might make you fall asleep more quickly, but your slumber will be more restless and less restorative. Alcohol sedates the brain activity that is vital for REM sleep, the most emotionally healing of sleep phases. In fact, in regular heavy drinkers and alcoholics, REM sleep is so stifled that many of them dream very little, which leads to daytime thinking difficulties.

Alcohol leaves you sleep-deprived and groggy, even if you think you had enough hours. If you drank enough to cause a hangover, then expect it to feel that much worse.

Unlike sleeping pills, which are of some use, alcohol is never a good sleeping aid. You need that REM to get the full restorative benefits of sleep (see pages 228–229).

Will Digital Devices Keep Me Awake?

Put the phone away if you want a good night's sleep, goes the modern mantra—but your body is too smart to be duped by a tiny screen into thinking it's daytime.

Gazing intently into the blaze of a digital screen deep into the night has long been identified as the enemy of restful sleep, especially in teenagers and young people, for whom sleep has an especially important role.

The theory goes that the blue-toned light from the backlit glow of a digital device tricks the body clock into thinking it is still daytime, pushing the body clock forward, delaying

53% OF PEOPLE IN THE **US ADMIT THEY CHECK** THEIR **PHONE LAST** THING AT **NIGHT**

WANT TO DIAL DOWN THE DIGITAL DAMAGE?

1

DO SOMETHING NONDIGITAL before bed—an activity that encourages the brain's "wandering" network will allow your body clock to work unhindered.

2

IF YOU MUST USE A DEVICE, avoid fast-paced apps—they'll trigger energizing, wakeful hormones.

3

NIGHT-LIGHT MODE with its dim, reddish light almost certainly won't improve your sleep, but it may be less annoying for a partner trying to drop off.

the melatonin gong, and thus making it more difficult to drift off.

The basis for this thinking is that blueish light—similar to the blue of a clear sky, and almost identical to the frequency of daylight that our aquatic ancestors would have seen when looking up through the ocean's waves—is the hue that the body clock is most sensitive to. The theory is right, but science reveals that the sleep-disrupting effect of digital blue light is likely overstated—your body is too clever to be "awoken" by such small screens; they're simply not bright enough to make the body clock think that it's daytime.

Furthermore, once you've nodded off, any danger of blue-light insomnia has largely passed. Should you wake up in the night and glance at a digital screen, any awakening effect from the light is minimal. In the middle of the night, the body's sleep cogs are already in full motion. A digital device isn't going to derail your sleep by tricking your body's wily timekeepers into believing night is day.

However, this doesn't mean that your devices are sleep-friendly. Those energizing stress hormones produced when playing a game, browsing online, or trawling social media are highly likely to override your sleep impulses and keep you wired long after bedtime.

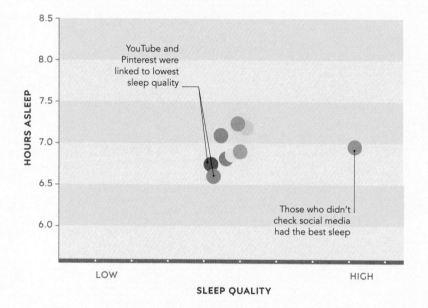

YouTube and Pinterest were linked to lowest sleep quality

Those who didn't check social media had the best sleep

HOURS ASLEEP

SLEEP QUALITY

LOW — HIGH

STIMULATING SOCIAL MEDIA

A large survey in the US compared people's rating of their quality of sleep with the social media apps they checked just before bed. All the apps were associated to some extent with poorer sleep, although it seemed that there was no effect on length of sleep. People who didn't check any social media reported by far the best quality sleep.

KEY

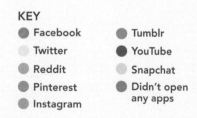

- Facebook
- Twitter
- Reddit
- Pinterest
- Instagram
- Tumblr
- YouTube
- Snapchat
- Didn't open any apps

What's the Best Way to Fall—and Stay—Asleep?

Good sleep can be worryingly hard to come by for many people. The three factors that most affect your chances of sweet dreams are temperature, light, and, above all, routine.

Since you're most vulnerable to threat when you're asleep, humans are programmed to drift off only when the coast is clear—and that's when we're calm and relaxed. Anxiety, worry, and any kind of trigger to your fight-or-flight response, whether it's fretting about an unpaid bill, a stressful deadline, or even dreading not being able to sleep, feeds your body a pulse of adrenaline, sabotaging good sleep by hurling the brain out of its relaxed state. Counting sheep or watching the clock just makes things worse—they switch on your brain's "watching" network, which delays sleep even more. Sleep will come easier if you ease your brain into its freewheeling "wandering" network by doing familiar, uncomplicated tasks, such as brushing your teeth.

Temperature and light are key to sleep. We know from studying hunter-gatherer communities, whose lifestyle has changed little in thousands of years, that humans naturally sleep a couple of hours after it gets dark and the air temperature has fallen. In line

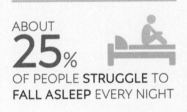

ABOUT
25%
OF PEOPLE **STRUGGLE** TO **FALL ASLEEP** EVERY NIGHT

SLEEP HYGIENE
The term "sleep hygiene" was coined by sleep scientists and simply means developing a positive, helpful sleep routine. All studies show that sticking to some basic, universal rules really can purify your sleep.

AVOID HEAVY MEALS in the evening. Like most body systems, your intestines slow down at night. Bloating the stomach can lead to indigestion, which will disturb sleep. A large meal can also prod the body clock into daytime, wakeful behavior.

ESTABLISH A ROUTINE. We learn by repetition, so by finding a routine in the hour or so before bed and sticking to it, you can become a pro sleeper. This could involve brushing your teeth, dimming the lights, taking a bath, or meditating.

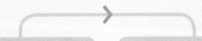

with this, your body clock winds down your alertness and body temperature. If your bedroom is too hot, you simply won't be able to sleep well because your core temperature is too high.

Absolute darkness is supremely soporific for both achieving sleep and staying in the land of zeds. It has taken Mother Nature 3.6 million years to teach us how to sleep, using the daylight-temperature partnership as fail-safe signals to our internal clock. Like a bewildered moth spiraling into a lantern, our brain wiring cannot reconcile bright light with night. Get as much daylight as you can during the day, but in the hour before bed, try turning off half of the lights in your home to help guide your brain home.

If you go camping, you will probably find that you fall into this natural rhythm within a day or two. Interestingly, when sleeping under the stars, morning larks and night owls tend to find their body clocks come a little closer together.

HALF-ASLEEP DUCKS AND DOLPHINS

Our brains need full, deep sleep, but that's not the case across the whole animal kingdom. For dolphins and other aquatic mammals who need to surface to breathe oxygen, only half of the brain sleeps at a time. Through the night, they keep one eye open and one half of their brain alert, before swapping sides to give the other half a rest.

Ducks use a similar strategy. Lining up for safety, the ducks at each end of the row sleep with one eye open and half of their brain alert. A predator can then be spotted by the half-sleeping sentries.

Even more impressive, newborn dolphins and orcas do not sleep at all for a whole month after birth, and nor do their mothers, who stay fully awake to keep both eyes on their offspring!

KEEP CONSISTENT HOURS. Go to bed and rise at the same times, even on the weekends. The body clock doesn't understand the five-day workweek and thrives on routine, which is closely tied with our safety-first instincts.

ALLOW SLEEP OPPORTUNITY. To have any hope of staying in "wandering" brain mode, sleep can't be rushed. Seven hours' sleep does not mean seven hours in bed. Allow yourself extra time—at least half an hour—to fall asleep.

DON'T LIE awake for hours—you'll train your brain to link bed with alertness. Get up and go to another room. Dim the lights and read or listen to music. Go back to bed when you feel sleepy, and repeat if you still can't sleep after 20 minutes.

Is Sleep Really That Important?

Sleep is a refreshing, healing tonic that nourishes and repairs body and mind. It's a daily prescription more powerful than the most expensive drugs—and it's free.

On the face of it, sleep is a ludicrous, dangerous waste of time, rendering you unproductive and, in a primal sense, unable to defend or nourish yourself. But make no mistake, sleep is no accident. Very soon after animal life emerged on planet Earth, sleep followed. Every animal that lives longer than a week sleeps in some way or another. If you live by the go-getter motto, "I'll sleep when I'm dead," then you can bet your bottom dollar that the fateful day will come sooner than you think.

Feeling ratty after a bad night? When you're sleep deprived, the emotional, impulsive brain regions explode with activity, making an otherwise amiable person crotchety, snappy, and more likely to hear a benign comment as a personal slight. Every mental health disorder and illness, bar none, has been linked with disordered sleep. Once, we thought that psychiatric disorders led to sleep problems. In reality, it's a two-way street, with lack of sleep contributing to mental ill-health, and those mental health issues making sleep even worse.

On average, people eat about 400 calories more a day when poorly slept. It's perhaps no surprise that obesity rates have sky-rocketed in line with our worsening sleep habits; many researchers are now convinced the worldwide obesity epidemic is rooted in so many of us going skinny on sleep. If you're trying to lose weight, being low on sleep will hamper your efforts. This is because in a sleep-deficient state, your body clings on to fat,

AFTER **POOR SLEEP, ACTIVITY** IN THE **IMPULSIVE REGIONS** OF THE **BRAIN RISES BY** **60**%

FURTHER QUESTIONS AFFECTED BY SLEEP

- Page 64–65: "How can I get the most from my working day?"
- Page 80: "Why do I feel hungry again so soon after breakfast?"
- Pages 132–133: "How can I improve my memory?"
- Pages 162–163: "What's the best way to build up muscle?"

believing lack of sleep means your life is under threat.

Lack of sleep also hits your immune system. After four hours' slumber, the following morning will see numbers of cancer-fighting cells depleted, making these essential defenders less able to ward off assaults. If you regularly don't sleep enough, your joints, muscles, and bones will ache, your arteries are more likely to fur up, and even your fertility is lowered. Sports injury rates are four times higher in those who sleep six hours per night, compared to those who enjoy nine hours.

FEWER COLDS AND COUGHS
Sleep supercharges the immune system, bolstering the body's ability to fight off seasonal infections.

BETTER WEIGHT MANAGEMENT
If you're exercising or on a diet, good sleep ensures your body will burn off excess fat instead of muscle.

IMPROVED MOOD
After a good night's sleep, levels of positive hormone serotonin rise, while anxiety-inducing hormones such as cortisol and adrenaline plummet.

HEALTHY BRAIN
During slow-wave sleep, tiny drainage canals in the brain called glymphatic channels wash away toxic sludge and molecular detritus. This nightly cleanup is vital for brain health and may prevent degenerative brain conditions such as Alzheimer's disease.

DECREASED HUNGER
Leptin, a powerful appetite-suppressing hormone, is released after a good night's sleep, keeping cravings in check.

FITTER BODY
Muscle strength is boosted by regularly sleeping well. The body repairs and strengthens during the deepest, slow-wave sleep.

BETTER MENTAL HEALTH
Sufficient rest and an established sleep routine help prevent the onset of mental illness and improve existing conditions.

THE BENEFITS OF SLEEP

How Do I Know How Much Sleep I Need?

The recommendation is at least seven hours, with about eight hours the optimum—but some people claim they need much less, or much more. This is what the science says.

Everyone is different, and the amount of sleep everyone needs can vary—but probably not as much as you think. A few people cope well and perform normally without the usual amount of sleep—waking at 5 a.m. every morning without flagging. Don't try to train yourself to be like them—it would be akin to trying to change your eye color. People who function well on four to six hours, rather than the usual eight, are usually born with a mutation in one of several wakefulness-controlling genes (with catchy names such as DEC2, ADRB1, or NPSR1, among many others). Whether such light sleepers eventually suffer the same ill health as others would from a lifetime's lack of sleep is as yet unknown.

Your body clock (see pages 22–23) controls when you feel like going to sleep and when you wake up. Listen to your body and go to sleep when you feel tired, and try to wake up naturally every day. Don't forget that naps count toward your daily total, and even a 20-minute snooze can be useful if you are flagging following a disturbed night. Also, be aware that the amount of sleep you need tends to gradually reduce as you age.

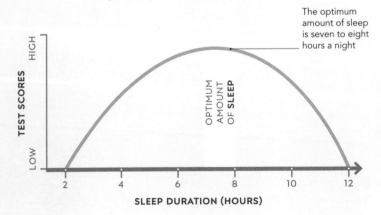

The optimum amount of sleep is seven to eight hours a night

TEST SCORES — HIGH / LOW

OPTIMUM AMOUNT OF SLEEP

SLEEP DURATION (HOURS)
2   4   6   8   10   12

FIND YOUR BALANCE
One study showed that people struggle to complete simple tests in the lab not only when they've had too little sleep but also when they've had too much!

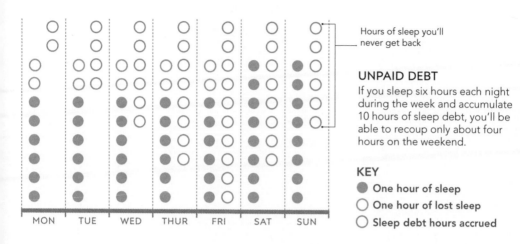

UNPAID DEBT
If you sleep six hours each night during the week and accumulate 10 hours of sleep debt, you'll be able to recoup only about four hours on the weekend.

KEY
● One hour of sleep
○ One hour of lost sleep
○ Sleep debt hours accrued

| MON | TUE | WED | THUR | FRI | SAT | SUN |

Can I Make Up for Lost Sleep on the Weekend?

You might look forward to sleeping in on the weekend, especially after a busy week. However, there's a limit to catching up on sleep. Some hours will be lost forever.

In some ways, sleep is like food. Starve yourself of its nourishment and your body will feast on it when next given the chance, refilling drained reserves.

After a night or two of poor rest, we will naturally sleep longer on subsequent nights. We accumulate a "sleep debt" that we carry until we can get decent shut-eye. Powerfully restorative to body and mind, it is slow-wave sleep that your body craves most when you've been burning the candle at both ends. In catch-up sleep, more time is spent in the slow-wave

stage, so you will experience fewer exciting dreams.

Unfortunately, the body can't fully recoup lost sleep, but that's not to say you shouldn't catch up on as much as you can. No matter how big the debt, you can normally manage only two or three extra hours over and above your normal nightly total, so sleeping in on the weekend can only claw back so much lost time. The "interest" you pay on sleep debt is poor long-term health, so it's vital to keep your sleep hours in the black as often as you can.

What Can I Do if I Can't Avoid Sleep Deprivation?

In these hyper-busy, time-poor days, it's tempting to try to get through by skimping on sleep. But be careful you don't sleepwalk into your own personal disaster.

Many people claim they can get by just fine with only four or five hours of sleep, and the demands of modern life sometimes require us to be alert and available 24/7. However, sleep deprivation is dangerous, and

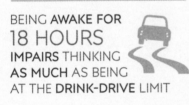

BEING **AWAKE FOR**
18 HOURS
IMPAIRS THINKING
AS MUCH AS BEING
AT THE **DRINK-DRIVE** LIMIT

perhaps the most sinister nature of it is that we don't realize just how tired we are. Termed "baseline resetting," we get so used to a fatigued existence that we think spending life wading against waves of tiredness is normal.

Your brain starts to glitch and you'll have momentary lapses—brief episodes, called "microsleeps," when you're completely unaware of the world. Your brain is so desperate to get some slow-wave sleep that it literally cuts the power. If you're reading a book, it's harmless—you'll reread the same sentence again—but if you're cruising down the highway, the consequences will be catastrophic. Someone who has slept for less than

four hours is a staggering 11 times more likely to be in a car crash than someone with eight hours of sleep. Planning a long drive and didn't sleep well last night? Leave the keys at home and catch a train instead.

Sometimes, there's no alternative to sleep deprivation—new parents and resident doctors are among those who simply have to get through it. (A study showed that resident doctors who worked 34-hour shifts made 460 percent more diagnostic mistakes.) Research is ongoing into the long-term effects of sleep deprivation, but it is clear that both physical and mental health are at risk for those who don't get sufficient sleep over a sustained period.

If you work very long shifts, try to claw back some sleep on rest days. If you can, plan demanding tasks for your first day back, when you are more rested. For new parents, grab sleep whenever your baby does—it may not be continuous, restful slumber, but those snatched minutes can accrue into a surprising amount of shut-eye.

> "With baseline resetting, your **tiredness becomes** the **norm** and you **no longer notice** your **low alertness** and **impaired judgment**."

How Can I Deal with Jet Lag?

Jet lag can be grim. Your body clock influences all your body systems, and the time it takes to adjust to new time zones depends on how far you've traveled.

Before aircraft could speed us around the globe, jet lag didn't exist—we traveled slowly enough for our bodies to adjust to gradually changing time zones. Jet lag happens when the body clock is out of step with the actual time, causing you to be in night mode when it is daytime (and vice versa).

Flying east is usually harder than flying west. Traveling east usually means you are catching up with the sun and so will arrive at a later hour than your body clock is expecting. Going to bed before your body is ready is not easy; cortisol levels haven't yet drooped and the melatonin message that the end of the day is nigh has not yet been sent. Flying westward is typically less torturous, because you have to stay up later—and that's far easier to do, both mentally and biologically.

Such is the command of the body clock, there is simply no way to avoid jet lag. After you've arrived at a different time zone, your internal clock will slide forward or backward by about one hour each day. So if your destination time is seven hours out of kilter with your home time, then expect it to take a full week before your body has fully adjusted into the new groove.

WANT TO **BEAT JET LAG?**

1
AVOID CAFFEINE AND ALCOHOL on the flight because these will make it more difficult to get into the groove of your destination time zone.

2
EAT MEALS AT THE TIME OF YOUR DESTINATION during your flight, to help the body clock harmonize with the new time zone.

3
GET INTO DAYLIGHT as early as possible and avoid wearing sunglasses so that you feed loud "wake-up!" messages to the brain. Even cloudy conditions will prod your body clock in the right direction.

4
SHUT OUT LIGHT later in the day—by wearing sunglasses and closing the curtains, you will blunt your body clock's drive to stay awake.

5
SLOG OUT THE REST OF THE DAY and try to stay awake until your new time zone's bedtime, to nudge your body clock into its new rhythm.

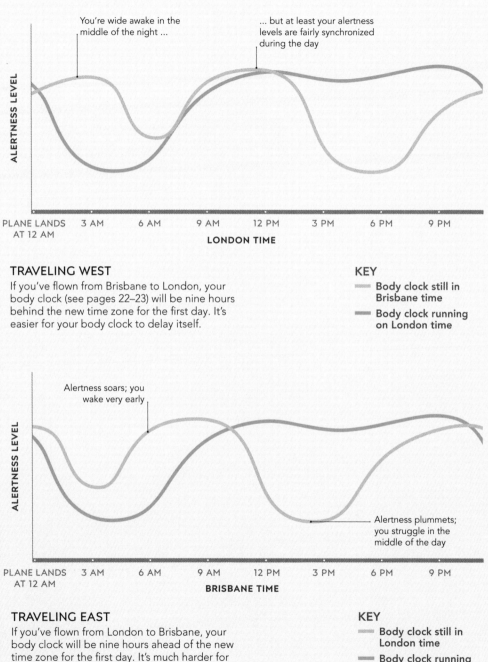

You're wide awake in the middle of the night ...

... but at least your alertness levels are fairly synchronized during the day

ALERTNESS LEVEL

PLANE LANDS AT 12 AM   3 AM   6 AM   9 AM   12 PM   3 PM   6 PM   9 PM

LONDON TIME

TRAVELING WEST

If you've flown from Brisbane to London, your body clock (see pages 22–23) will be nine hours behind the new time zone for the first day. It's easier for your body clock to delay itself.

KEY
Body clock still in Brisbane time

Body clock running on London time

Alertness soars; you wake very early

ALERTNESS LEVEL

Alertness plummets; you struggle in the middle of the day

PLANE LANDS AT 12 AM   3 AM   6 AM   9 AM   12 PM   3 PM   6 PM   9 PM

BRISBANE TIME

TRAVELING EAST

If you've flown from London to Brisbane, your body clock will be nine hours ahead of the new time zone for the first day. It's much harder for your body clock to advance itself.

KEY
Body clock still in London time

Body clock running on Brisbane time

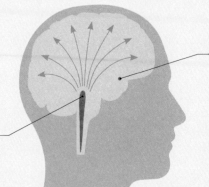

The VLPO is a tiny region neighboring the hypothalamus

The RAS is a network of connections sprouting from the brainstem

BODY HICCUP
When you're awake, the RAS rules the roost, but come bedtime, when the VLPO is pumped up by the tiredness hormone adenosine, it eventually takes control.

Why Do I Get Sleep Jerks?

The room is dark, the duvet warm, and the mattress soft ... then for no apparent reason, you are jolted wide awake as if hit by lightning. What's going on?

Taking place in the lightest stages of sleep, these momentary quakes are called "hypnagogic jerks." Usually they involve a falling sensation but can also be an imagined noise, or a flash of light. Around 70–80 percent of people say they experience them, and they happen because of a wrestling match between the drive to stay awake and the pulling force of sleep. Wearing the red belt in this bout is the fleet-footed reticular activating system, or the RAS, fighting to keep you awake. It faces off against the sleepy pillow-yearning region, the ventrolateral preoptic nucleus, or the VLPO. Although smaller, the VLPO is destined to win, but a jerk happens when

the struggling RAS lands a brief heavy blow. One theory suggests that sleep jerks are a survival relic handed down from our tree-dwelling ancestors. As your muscles relax in the early stages of sleep, your primate brain jolts you awake when it senses you are about to tumble out of the tree.

They're completely harmless— assuming that a flying arm doesn't land on a loved one. They are as common in the well rested as in those with sleep problems and become less frequent as you get older. There is little evidence, but some claim that reducing caffeine intake and late-night exercise reduces the occurrence of sleep jerks.

Why Do I Talk in My Sleep?

If you are prone to holding conversations while fast asleep, rest easy: your subconscious isn't leaking your deepest secrets, and you're not unwell.

Surprisingly, you don't sleep talk during vivid dreams—your jabberings actually arise out of the tranquility of slow-wave sleep. Similar to sleep jerks, sleep talking (termed "somniloquy") seems to be a break in the veil of sleep. During deep sleep, the brain's VLPO region is at the helm, releasing two powerful substances—GABA and glycine—that paralyze you. Only a few movements slip through the net of paralysis, such as rolling over (which seems to be the body's protection against getting bed sores). Moans, laughter, or speech also quite frequently burst through this paralysis. Similarly, sleepwalking also arises from deep sleep—contrary to what many people think, sleepwalkers are not acting out a dream.

These escapees from the paralysis straitjacket are nothing to worry about. Sleepwalking is common in young children, and most people grow out of it by adulthood, in line with the maturing of our sleep-controlling brain systems. Nevertheless, sleepwalking runs in families, and 2–3 percent of adults sleepwalk from time to time. If you've been drinking alcohol or are sleep deprived, you're more likely to go wandering in the night. Stress and anxiety also weaken the VLPO's grip, making sleep talking more likely. People suffering from post-traumatic stress disorder (PTSD) are predisposed to voicing nocturnal narratives.

People fear that waking a sleepwalker is dangerous. It may be disorientating, but it's in no way life-threatening. The person is in deep sleep and will likely wake with a start, just as if you shook them awake in bed.

60% OF **PEOPLE TALK** IN THEIR **SLEEP—SWEARING** IS SURPRISINGLY **COMMON!**

Why Do I Snore and How Can I Stop?

Snoring is a strange side effect of floppy muscles during deep sleep that is annoying to many, usually harmless, but is sometimes dangerous.

Like bad breath, most of us don't know we snore until someone tells us. And it's common: around four in 10 men and a quarter of women do it. Snoring occurs in the deepest stages of sleep when your muscles are at their floppiest: tissues holding the roof of the mouth and tongue in place sag so much that they dangle in front of the windpipe. With each breath, they flap and vibrate noisily, like a door banging in the breeze. If you have swollen tonsils, a throat infection, or hay fever, this will inflame throat tissues and narrow your airway, making snoring even worse. Generally, the larger you are, the louder the snoring, while some people are born with a nose or jaw shape that means they can deliver thunderous snorts at night.

Useless anti-snoring aids abound, including rings worn on the little finger that claim to stimulate "acupressure sites" to prevent snoring. Snorers and their partners are not without hope for more peace, though. The type of aid to choose depends on whether the noise mainly comes from the nasal passageways or a constricted throat.

IN A UK SURVEY, 12% OF RESPONDENTS **CITED SNORING** AS ONE OF THE **REASONS** FOR **DIVORCING**

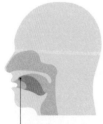

Push the tip of your tongue against the roof of your mouth and slide it backward 20 times

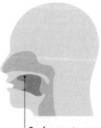

Suck your tongue upward so its entire top surface lies against the roof of your mouth 20 times

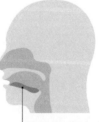

Force the back of your tongue down against the floor of your mouth while keeping the tip of your tongue in contact with your bottom front teeth 20 times

SNORE NO MORE
If practiced every day, these exercises strengthen the muscles around the airways to reduce snoring and improve sleep quality.

Chin straps and mouth guards are designed to stop mouth breathing or lift the jaw to allow airflow. These can help mouth-based snorers, although may be so uncomfortable they affect the snorer's ability to sleep.

Nasal strips and tubes can help nasal snorers by widening the nostrils to reduce turbulence. Nasal sprays are scientifically proven to expand the airways and reduce the din, although steroid-based sprays can affect your sleep quality by impairing REM sleep. In severe cases, surgery to remove tissue at the back of the throat offers a solution for very problematic snoring.

However, before trying a human-made remedy, there are simple, cost-free changes you can make that are proven to deliver a quieter night.

WANT TO CALL TIME ON YOUR SNORING?

1
AVOID ALCOHOL OR SEDATIVE MEDICATION— both will relax throat muscles more and worsen the problem.

2
DON'T SLEEP ON YOUR BACK—in this position, the tongue and palate vibrate against the back of the throat. Side sleeping is the best position for snorers.

3
IF YOU ARE OVERWEIGHT, shedding even a couple of pounds can ease enough pressure on the airways to allow for quieter breathing.

OSA, THE NOT-SO-SILENT KILLER

Snoring isn't generally harmful to the snorer's health. However, there's a chance that snoring may be your body's distress call, signaling a life-threatening condition called obstructive sleep apnea (OSA). This is when the throat muscle tissues sag so much at night that they completely block the airway. With a cough and a splutter you'll awaken, then drift back to deep sleep, at which point the muscles relax once again and the splutter-wake-sleep cycle continues.

OSA can be deadly. Repeated brief suffocations through the night wreak havoc on body systems and cause the memory-storing hippocampus to shrivel. You're also at higher risk of obesity, type 2 diabetes, high blood pressure, heart attacks, and mental illness.

Around 5 percent of adults in developed countries have OSA, but 85 percent of sufferers are unaware of it. Very effective treatment is available once a person is diagnosed—the hallmark of OSA is feeling exhausted and unrefreshed after sleep. Other clues include nodding off at the drop of a hat in the daytime, being overweight, and unusually loud snoring. See a doctor without delay if this sounds like you.

Why Do I Get Night Terrors or Sleep Paralysis?

For many, these horrifying nighttime visitations are all too real. Night terrors and sleep paralysis are both disturbing, but they originate from different stages of the sleep cycle.

If you've ever woken in the night, unable to move and aware of something sinister nearby, then you've experienced sleep paralysis—the flip of sleepwalking. Your brain has awoken, but your body is asleep. You can't move or speak because your sleep centers continue to immobilize your limbs, mistakenly thinking you are still in dreaming (REM) sleep. Your eyes are free to roam, and the reticular activating system has turned the lights on upstairs, but the flow of natural muscle sedatives has not yet been stemmed. Around a fifth of adults experience this horrible but harmless phenomenon. Crucially, this frightening parasomnia (the term used for disorders in the sleep cycle) happens during light REM sleep.

In contrast, night terrors arise from the slow-wave stage of sleep. The brain has tried to rise from the depths of deep sleep but can't quite surface. The eyes are open, but the mind is sloshing around in largely dreamless, slow-wave sleep. For reasons no one yet understands, the fear and anxiety pathways get caught in a loop and you might scream the house down.

Resolution, as for all parasomnias, can often be found in good sleep hygiene (see pages 226–227).

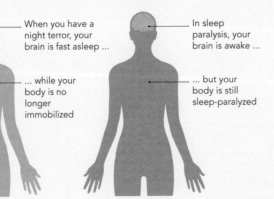

When you have a night terror, your brain is fast asleep ...

... while your body is no longer immobilized

In sleep paralysis, your brain is awake ...

... but your body is still sleep-paralyzed

SLEEP MALFUNCTIONS

In sleep paralysis, the time lapse between the brain waking and your body freeing itself from paralysis can be a few seconds or several minutes. Roles are reversed when it comes to night terrors—and they can also last several minutes.

"

During sleep
paralysis, as your
thinking mind
casts around to make
sense of the body's
immobility, terrifying
imaginings and
hallucinations
can take hold.

"

Does Dreaming Make Me More Creative?

Dreaming is the brain's go-to sandbox for playing around with unusual ideas and trying out solutions that our logic-driven conscious brain would dismiss out of hand.

Not every problem has a straightforward solution. Often, predicaments or dilemmas need creative, lateral thought and leaps of logic—and your methodical frontal lobe brain regions aren't always suited to these tasks. When you dream, however, your emotional centers play by different rules. Like a police detective's investigation board, experiences, places, and faces can be "pinned up," then rearranged and strung together in many different ways to reveal previously unnoticed connections and hidden solutions.

After a day or evening spent trying to master something new—be it a video game, a musical instrument, or taking up a new sport—you'll likely notice that these daytime efforts leak into your nocturnal mental wanderings. This ability is crucial to learning and developing new skills, and to weave these new experiences into your existing mental meshwork, effectively lining up the cellular cables so that everything

Thalamus blocks incoming sounds or feelings from body

Parietal cortex is inactive, disabling physical movement while you dream

Rational prefrontal cortex is powered down, allowing dreams to break all the laws of logic

Visual cortex conjures vivid imagery, drawing from your visual memory store

Amygdala supercharges your dreams with emotions

THE DREAMING BRAIN

Your dreams are wacky and weird because the sensible and logical prefrontal cortex is completely switched off, allowing your brain to creatively freestyle.

BRAIN CROSS SECTION

Hippocampus is active, remixing memories to serve as a basis for your dreams runs smoothly. This may be another reason babies do so much REM sleeping—their new world is full of new experiences, so their dreaming brains have to work overtime to assimilate them.

When your brain is firing in its most relaxed state (see page 70), creative ideas and out-of-the-box thinking are more common—and these abilities are supercharged during REM sleep.

IN A STUDY, **30**% OF **PEOPLE** SAID THEY REGULARLY **SOLVE PROBLEMS** IN THEIR **DREAMS**

Without a doubt, dreams are a hotbed of creativity out of which musical motifs and artistic ideas can bubble. Paul McCartney's *Yesterday* and *Let It Be* are just two of the countless examples of songs birthed in a dreamscape. Surrealist painter Salvador Dalí used to eat sea urchins in dark chocolate sauce before bed, hoping that it would make his dreams more bizarre, but science has yet to back up his logic.

You'll be more likely to remember your creative inspirations if you wake from REM sleep (see pages 18–19). And there's plenty of evidence of a strong link between better mental abilities and getting good REM sleep, especially in childhood.

MENDELEEV'S ATOMIC DREAM

Perhaps the most famous dream-induced eureka moment came in the late 1860s. Russian chemist Dmitri Mendeleev was obsessed with the scientific mystery of the day, which was trying to figure out a pattern to the chemical elements—the gases, metals, and other pure substances out of which everything is made.

Mendeleev made himself a set of cards, one for each of the 63 known elements, recording their qualities and atomic mass. In every spare moment, he would compulsively shuffle and lay out the cards, hoping that he could discover some organization to every type of atom. Red-eyed from failure and sleepless nights, he went to bed, and on February 17, 1869, wrote:

"I saw in a dream a table, where all the elements fell into place as required. Awakening, I immediately wrote it down on a piece of paper. Only in one place did a correction later seem necessary."

Mendeleev's breakthrough—the periodic table—was earth-shattering for science. Not only did he uncover the code, but he even left gaps for undiscovered elements, predicting what these mystery atoms would be like with prophetlike accuracy.

Do My Dreams Mean Anything?

Dreams are "you" in your purest form, without the distractions of the world. Why we dream is disputed, but whatever the reason, your brain is getting a great workout.

It seems that there is something of a "dream switch" in the brain. About 90 minutes after slipping out of the conscious world, the brain jolts awake, making your eyes dart back and forth as if watching a TV show projected on the inside of the eyelids. The instant we start dreaming, a part of the brain known as the posterior cortical hot zone "ignites". Straddling various visual, sensory, and emotional parts of the brain, this network integrates information from these areas. When flicked on, the "hot zone" indicates that you are having a conscious experience and are dreaming. You are seeing and feeling—totally immersed within your inner virtual reality.

Dreaming has meaning and value from the brain's point of view. If you are deprived of REM sleep, then the following night you will dream longer and more vividly as your brain claims back the missed REM sleep.

In REM sleep, dreams often feel more intense than real life. When scanned in an MRI machine, the emotional parts of the brain are 30

ABOUT **65%** OF DREAMS ARE FILLED WITH **SADNESS**, AND **ONLY**

20%

WITH **HAPPINESS**

percent more active during dreaming than when awake. Across culture and creed, dreams dramatize universal human wishes, fears, and concerns—often mutating a mundane situation into a worst-case scenario.

Dreams are a paradox; your surreal nighttime imaginings are fascinating and profoundly meaningful to you but dull or just plain weird to others. The purpose and meaning of dreams are as perplexing as their contents. Lurid or bizarre dreams are the ones that stick in the memory, but studies show that they make up only a tiny proportion of the whole—around 1–2 percent. Almost all our dreams are mundane and sound entirely unremarkable when we attempt to describe them to someone else.

Threat simulation
Your mind is figuring out how to deal with obstacles that you might face when awake. Fleeing from lions, battling aliens, or escaping a burning building—such dreams are rehearsals for events that might happen in the waking world.

The psychoanalytic theory
Sigmund Freud theorized in 1900 that dreams are disguised fulfillments of repressed wishes. The detail of his ideas is considered off the mark from a scientific standpoint today, but this was nevertheless a watershed in understanding that dreams come from within us.

Fear reduction
This idea builds on the threat simulation theory: if you face your fears in the safety of your dream, you might worry less and extinguish that fear in your waking life. This theory also explains how dreams might "fail," resulting in a nightmare.

Memory consolidation
Slow-wave sleep (nREM) has been proven to strengthen memories, and this theory posits that dreaming in the REM stage of sleep is the brain's effort to knit together connections between memories that wouldn't be made when you were awake.

Activation-synthesis
Dreaming is simply a by-product of an energetic brain and an imaginative mind. Essentially, dreams are freewheeling thoughts and emotions that have no purpose other than to keep the brain ticking over when the lights are out.

Future prediction
The ever-popular and far-fetched theory that dreams predict the future is practically impossible to investigate scientifically. In the 1970s, a UK newspaper invited readers to send in their dreams, and, over the next 15 years, the science editor tried to link them to real-life events. He couldn't.

WHY DO WE DREAM?
There is no shortage of theories as to precisely why we dream, perhaps because such theories are so difficult for sleep scientists to test and prove one way or the other. Regardless of the reason, we do know that dreaming is beneficial to mental and physical health.

Glossary

Adenosine
A neurotransmitter that promotes sleep. It is lowest in the morning and increases with each waking hour.

Adipose cells
Your body fat is made up of these cells—they can be the white or brown type.

Adrenaline
Powerful hormone that boosts heart and breathing rates; main player in the body's fight-or-flight response.

Amygdala
Almond-shaped cluster of cells in the brain's limbic system. Involved in threat detection, triggering fear responses, formimg emotional memories, and strengthening learning.

Antioxidants
Chemicals in the body and in foodstuffs that neutralize waste known as free radicals.

Basal ganglia
Brain structure that controls habitual, autopilot behaviors (your procedural memory).

Body clock
Also known as circadian rhythm, a natural body system that controls sleepiness and wakefulness over a day. Mainly controlled by the SCN.

Brain circuitry
Interlinked brain cells that carry messages and trigger body functions.

Brain-derived neurotrophic factor (BDNF)
Protective protein produced by brain cells; helps you to think faster and new brain cells to grow.

Carbohydrates (carbs)
Key nutrients including sugars and starch; important in energy production.

Cerebellum
Large, wrinkled structure on the brain's underside; important in smooth movement, balance, and procedural memory.

Cholecystokinin (CCK)
Gut hormone that is released when the first part of the intestine is full of food. Makes food stay in stomach longer, reduces appetite, and makes you feel full and sleepy after meals.

Chronotype
An individual's body-clock timing, which controls the sleep-wake cycle.

"Concentrating" network
See Executive control network.

Confirmation bias
Tendency to take in information in a way that confirms what you already believe.

Cortisol
One of the stress hormones. Increases blood sugar and blood pressure and calms immune system.

Default mode network
Interlinked system of brain areas, active when your mind is wandering and not working toward a particular goal. The brain's most relaxed state.

Dopamine
The body's main "reward" hormone and neurotransmitter. Imbues strong feelings of satisfaction and elation.

Dunning-Kruger effect
Tendency in most people to overestimate their own abilities and performance in a particular area.

Endorphins
Hormones produced in the brain that numb pain and cause euphoria. The body's "natural painkillers".

Estrogen
The main female sex hormone, which prompts female sexual development. Present in males in lower levels.

Executive control network
Interlinked brain circuitry in the frontal lobes. Active when you concentrate, make decisions, and solve problems.

Fiber
Nutrient found in plant-based foods that your body can't digest or absorb. Helps other foods pass through the gut.

Fight-or-flight response
A collection of bodily responses that are triggered as soon as we feel threatened.

Fluoride
Chemical added to toothpastes—reduces decay by strengthening the enamel coating of the teeth.

Fovea
Tiny pit at the back of the eye where our clearest vision comes from. Densely packed with cone cells (color vision sensors).

Free radicals
Unstable toxic substances produced in the body as part of normal wear and tear. They cause damage known as "oxidative stress."

FTO
Gene that regulates the amount of dopamine released when you eat and, therefore, the pleasure you get from food.

GABA
Mood-regulating neurotransmitter chemical that calms brain activity.

Ghrelin
The "hunger" hormone, released when your stomach is empty. Triggers an increase in appetite.

Glucagon
A "sugar-police" hormone released by the pancreas. When blood sugar is low, glucagon triggers the release of more sugar from body's stores.

Glutamate
Mood-regulating neurotransmitter that increases brain activity in certain areas.

Glycogen
The body's main store of carbohydrates, mostly in muscles and liver. Made up of chemical chains of glucose that can be broken down quickly.

Habit hub
See Basal ganglia.

Hippocampus
Inch-long, slug-shaped structure nestled by the limbic system. Stores, processes, and retrieves memories.

Hormones
Signaling molecules produced by glands and tissues. They are carried throughout the body by the blood, to trigger and regulate body processes.

Hypnagogic jerks
Sudden muscle spasms when you're on the brink of sleep, linked to a falling sensation.

Hypothalamus
Pea-sized area in the brain that regulates temperature, appetite, sex drive, and produces many of the main hormones.

Limbic system
Group of brain structures that contain the amygdala, hippocampus, and hypothalamus. Deals with emotions and memories.

Melanin
Natural UV-blocking pigment responsible for your skin tone and hair color.

Melatonin
One of the body's "sleep" hormones, released mainly from the brain's pineal gland.

Migrating motor complex
Regular pattern of contraction in your gut muscles between meals. Clears undigested food through your system.

Morning larks
People whose body clocks are biased toward waking early.

Also known as "early chronotypes."

Myelin tissue
Substance made of fats and proteins, which encases the long "tails" of nerve cells and helps nerve impulses travel rapidly and efficiently.

Neurotransmitters
Messaging substances in the brain that pass information between nerve cells. Also known as "brain hormones."

Neurons
The main brain cells that transmit electrical impulses and form brain circuits.

Night owls
People whose body clocks are biased to waking late and being energized in the evening. Also known as "late chronotypes."

Noradrenaline
Stress hormone and neurotransmitter. Increases heart rate and gets you ready for "fight-or-flight."

Nucleus accumbens
The brain's "pleasure hot spot"—releases dopamine, which can "reward" addictive behavior.

Orienting response
A survival reflex that prompts your attention by sudden sounds or movements.

Oxytocin
Hormone and neurotransmitter produced by the hypothalamus that fosters attachment and social bonding.

Parietal cortex
Upper region of the brain from where muscles are controlled and bodily sensations are felt. Important in sense of space and ability to navigate.

Pituitary gland
Pea-sized "master gland" at the base of the brain. Many of its hormones activate other glands and organs.

Postprandial somnolence
"Food coma"—the onset of sleepiness after eating. Caused by hormones such as cholecystokinin.

Prefrontal cortex
Area within frontal lobe that contains the circuitry most responsible for the brain's "executive" functions—its thinking.

Procedural memory
Scientific term for "muscle memory"—centered in the cerebellum and associated with habitual behaviors that require little conscious thought.

Protein
Key nutrient used in tissue repair, muscle growth, and hormone production. Most plentiful in meat, eggs, soybeans, and nuts.

Reticular activating system
(RAS) Brain network that controls whether we are awake and alert or asleep.

REM and nREM sleep
REM is the rapid eye movement stage of sleep, when the brain is as active as when awake and may be dreaming. During nREM (non-REM) sleep, brain activity is calmer and more organized.

Salience network
The "watching" network of the brain's circuitry. Triggered by distraction, it makes us vigilant to sudden changes and prepares us for action.

Saturated fats
Fats that are typically solid at room temperature. High intake leads to atherosclerosis—furring up of arteries.

Serotonin
Neurotransmitter that plays a role in happiness and well-being.

Sleep inertia
Grogginess typically felt when roused from deep sleep.

Spatial cortex
See Parietal cortex.

Starch
Carbohydrate found in plant-based foods such as potatoes, corn, and rice, which is broken down into sugars.

Stress response
Sequence of body changes that happen when put under threat. The fight-or-flight response is one part of the stress response.

Temporal lobe
Large area in the brain containing the limbic system. Important in memory, language, and vision.

Testosterone
The main male sex hormone. Increases sex drive, aggression, and muscle growth. Prompts male sexual development. Present in females in lower levels.

Trans fat
Very unhealthy type of fat, synthesized from unsaturated fats and used in some processed foods.

Unsaturated fat
Fats that are typically liquid at room temperature. Found in fish and plant oils and essential for good health.

Vasopressin
Calming hormone and neurotransmitter produced in the hypothalamus. Works alongside oxytocin to encourage people to bond.

VLPO
Ventrolateral preoptic nucleus—a tiny brain area close to the hypothalamus, it releases neurotransmitters that encourage sleep.

"Wandering" network
See Default mode network.

"Watching" network
See Salience network.

Index

Data credits

The publisher would like to thank the following for their kind permission to reproduce their data:
(Key: a-above; b-below/bottom; c-centre; f-far; l-left; r-right; t-top)

13 D. Bruck & D.L. Pisani, "The effects of sleep inertia on decision-making performance", *J Sleep Res*, 1999, 8(2):95–103.
doi:10.1046/j.1365-2869.1999.00150.x.
13 P. Tassi & A. Muzet, "Sleep inertia", *Sleep Med Rev*, 2000, 4(4):341–353.
doi:10.1053/smrv.2000.0098.
14 M. Terman & J. Terman, "Light Therapy for Seasonal and Nonseasonal Depression: Efficacy, Protocol, Safety, and Side Effects", *CNS Spectrums*, 2005, 10(8):647–663.
doi:10.1017/S1092852900019611, reproduced with permission. (b)
23 B.C. Koch et al., "Circadian sleep-wake rhythm disturbances in end-stage renal disease", *Nat Rev Nephrol*, 2009, 5(7):407–16.
doi:10.1038/nrneph.2009.8.
(melatonin and cortisol data).
23 Copyright 2004 National Sleep Foundation – www.sleepfoundation.org.
25 Adapted from: G. Zerbini & M. Merrow, "Time to learn: How chronotype impacts education", *Psych J*, 2017, 6(4):263–276.
doi:10.1002/pchj.178.
30 T. Walsh et al., "Fluoride toothpastes of different concentrations for preventing dental caries", *Cochrane Database of Systematic Reviews*, 2019, Issue 3, Art. No.: CD007868.
doi:10.1002/14651858.CD007868.pub3. (bl)
36 H. Isaksson et al., "High-fiber rye diet increases ileal excretion of energy and macronutrients compared with low-fiber wheat diet independent of meal frequency in ileostomy subjects", *Food Nutr Res*, 2013, 57(1). (b)
44 E.E. Helander et al., "Weight Gain over the Holidays in Three Countries", *N Engl J Med*, 2016, 375(12):1200–1202.
doi:10.1056/NEJMc1602012. (b)
53 B. Clark et al. (CTS, Department of Geography and Environmental Management, UWE, Bristol), "How commuting affects subjective wellbeing", *Transportation*, 2019, 1–29.
55 Adapted from: P. Parthasarathi et al., "Network Structure and Travel Time Perception", *PLoS ONE*, 2013, 8(10):e77718.
doi:10.1371/journal.pone.0077718

62–63 L. Nummenmaa et al., "Bodily maps of emotions", *Proc Natl Acad Sci USA*, 2014, 111(2):646-651.
doi:10.1073/pnas.1321664111. (b)
78 Adapted from: S.J. Ritchie et al., "Sex Differences in the Adult Human Brain: Evidence from 5216 UK Biobank Participants", *Cereb Cortex*, 2018, 28(8):2959–2975.
doi:10.1093/cercor/bhy109. (b)
81 M.M. Perrigue et al., "Higher Eating Frequency Does Not Decrease Appetite in Healthy Adults", *J Nutr*, 2016, 146(1):59–64.
doi:10.3945/jn.115.216978. (t)
90 C.R. Mahoney et al., "The Acute Effects of Meals on Cognitive Performance" in HR Lieberman et al., "Nutrition, brain, and behaviour", *Nutr Neurosci*, 2005, 73–91 (p31).
doi:10.1201/9780203564554.ch6. (b)
97 WHO, "WHO calls on countries to reduce sugars intake among adults and children", press release, 2015, who.int/mediacentre/news/releases/2015/sugar-guideline/en/, accessed Jun 2020. (c)
99 Adapted from: D.R. Reed & A.H. McDaniel, "The human sweet tooth", *BMC Oral Health*, 2006, 6(1):S17.
doi:10.1186/1472-6831-6-S1-S17.
106 A. Dijksterhuis et al., "On Making the Right Choice: The Deliberation-Without-Attention Effect", *Science*, 2006, 311(5763):1005–1007.
doi:10.1126/science.1121629.
123 C.M. Alberini & A. Travaglia (Society for Neuroscience), "Infantile Amnesia: A Critical Period of Learning to Learn and Remember", *J Neurosci*, 2017, 37(24):5783–5795.
doi:10.1523/JNEUROSCI.0324-17.2017. (b)
138 J.K. Hartshorne & L.T. Germine, "When does cognitive functioning peak? The asynchronous rise and fall of different cognitive abilities across the life span", *Psychol Sci*, 2015, 26(4):433–443.
doi:10.1177/0956797614567339. (b)
156 L. Cipryan et al., "Acute and Post-Exercise Physiological Responses to High-Intensity Interval Training in Endurance and Sprint Athletes", *J Sports Sci Med*, 2017, 16(2):219–229. (b)
164 D.H. Wasserman, "Four grams of glucose", *Am J Physiol Endocrinol Metab*, 2009, 296(1):E11-E21.
doi:10.1152/ajpendo.90563.2008, fig.2. (tr)
166 A. Puce et al., "Neural Bases for Social Attention in Healthy Humans", in *The Development of Social Attention in Human Infants*, 2015, pp93–127.
doi:10.1007/978-3-319-21368-2_4,fig.4.1. (b)

167 S. Brinkhues et al., "Socially isolated individuals are more prone to have newly diagnosed and prevalent type 2 diabetes mellitus: The Maastricht study", *BMC Public Health*, 2017, 17(955).
doi:10.1186/s12889-017-4948-6 (cl).
174 C. Wyart et al., "Smelling a Single Component of Male Sweat Alters Levels of Cortisol in Women", *J Neurosci*, 2007, 27(6):1261-1265.
doi:10.1523/JNEUROSCI.4430-06.2007.
Copyright 2007 Society for Neuroscience (clb).
185 A. Weiss et al., "Midlife crisis in great apes, *PNAS*, 2012, 109(49):19949–19952.
doi:10.1073/pnas.1212592109.
186 J.K. MacCormack & K.A. Lindquist, "Feeling hangry? When hunger is conceptualized as emotion", *Emotion*, 2019, 19(2):301–319.
doi:10.1037/emo0000422. (b)
189 CDC.
207 Adapted from: L. Castaldo et al., "Red Wine Consumption and Cardiovascular Health", *Molecules*, 2019, 24:3626. (tr)
207 K. Middleton Fillmore et al., "Moderate alcohol use and reduced mortality risk: Systematic error in prospective studies", *Addict Res Theory*, 2006, 14(2):101–132.
doi:10.1080/16066350500497983. (tcb)
221 Adapted from: B.J. Brown et al., "A Neural Basis for Contagious Yawning", *Curr Biol*, 2017, 27(17):2713–2717.e2.
doi:10.1016/j.cub.2017.07.062.
221 A.G. Guggisberg et al., "Why do we yawn? The importance of evidence for specific yawn-induced effects", *Neurosci Biobehav Rev*, 2011, 35(5):1302–1304.
doi:10.1016/j.neubiorev.2010.03.008.
222 K.J. Brower, "Alcohol's effects on sleep in alcoholics", *Alcohol Res Health*, 2001, 25(2):110–125.
223 T. Roehrs & T. Roth, "Sleep, sleepiness, and alcohol use", *Alcohol Res Health*, 2001, 25(2):101–109. (t)
230 C.J. Wild et al., "Dissociable effects of self-reported daily sleep duration on high-level cognitive abilities", *Sleep*, 2018, 41(12):zsy182.
doi:10.1093/sleep/zsy182, fig.3.
235 Copyright 2004 National Sleep Foundation – www.sleepfoundation.org.

To access the complete list of source materials, studies, and research supporting the text in this book, visit:
www.dk.com/lybl-biblio

ABOUT THE AUTHOR

Dr. Stuart Farrimond is a science and health writer, presenter, and communicator. He is also a trained medical doctor and teacher, and his writing appears in both the national and international press, including *New Scientist*, *The Independent*, and *The Washington Post*. He makes regular appearances on TV, radio, and at public events, and he presents a weekly radio science show. His widely publicized research spans a huge variety of topics. Stuart is also the author of DK's *The Science of Cooking* and *The Science of Spice*.

ACKNOWLEDGMENTS

Author acknowledgments
This book is dedicated to the many friends, family members, and colleagues who have shown such unwavering love and support through our darkest days. The scope of this book is so outrageously broad that no one person has a brain large enough to answer all the questions unaided. I am, therefore, indebted to the international all-star cast of experts and academics who have freely given their time to support this project—answering my questions and reading my drafts. At both the start and end of the book, sleep expert Dr. Neil Stanley has tirelessly explained the mysteries of sleep, magicking up research papers that put many a head-scratching problem to bed. Although only hinted at in the book, there exists a blazing argument over the nature of seasonal affective disorder (SAD, or "winter blues"), and several premier league players kindly gave me their angle: Assoc. Prof. Stuart Pierson (Clinical Neurosciences, John Radcliffe Hospital, Oxford, UK), Dr. Manuel Spitschan (Oxford, UK), Prof. Steven LoBello (Auburn University, Montgomery, Alabama), and Prof. Anna Wirz-Justice (University of Basel, Switzerland). When it came to being clean on brushing teeth and dental science, Prof. Martin Addy (University of Bristol, UK), Prof. Damien Walmsley (University of Birmingham, UK,) and Prof. Philippe Hujoel (University of Washington, Seattle, Washington), helped me unpick the dirty myths. Hosts of the award-winning podcast *Minding the Brain*, Dr. Jim Davies and Dr. Kim Hellemans shared their thoughts on the evils (or not) of smartphone use. Assoc. Prof. Jenny Visser (Erasmus MC, Rotterdam, the Netherlands) and researcher Kasiphak Kaikaew helped me clear the air on the science of why women and men feel the heat differently. Prof. Alfonso Abizaid (Carleton University, Ottawa, Canada) helped make sure I had got everything gut-related in order, while Prof. James Betts (University of Bath, UK) repeatedly flexed his academic might in the great breakfast debate, and also later in sports nutrition research. Prof. Mark Sullman (University of Nicosia, Cyprus) and Dr. Amanda Stephens (Monash University,

Victoria, Australia) have dedicated much of their careers to understanding road rage. They shared their insights with me so that we can all see a little less red when behind the wheel. Assoc. Prof. Tamara Hew-Butler (Oakland University, Michigan) kindly poured out her knowledge on what science says about how much we should drink when on the go. On the exciting and baffling new science of brain networks, Assoc. Prof. Lucina Uddin (University of Miami, Florida) gave me an excellent heads-up on her research. And as the summer sun pounded, Professor Emeritus Brian Diffey (University of Newcastle, UK) shed some light on his life's work on the science of sun exposure. Special thanks also to radio presenter and friend Graham Seaman, who came to our rescue when we were wanting to make scary sounds look good.

I thank Dawn Henderson and Mary-Clare Jerram for welcoming me so warmly into the DK books fold. You both shared my vision for *Live Your Best Life* and stuck by me when an angry brain tumor decided to lay waste to well-made plans. My agent, Jonny Pegg, has similarly been a stalwart throughout. Senior Editor Rona Skene, who has waded through my writing from day one, has been ever encouraging. Frankie Piscitelli is our editing super trooper who was parachuted in for the final push. It has been an absolute joy to work with you.

It would be remiss of me not to give a most monumental thank you to my wife, Grace—the most fantastic wife a man could ever hope for.

Publisher acknowledgments
DK would like to thank John Friend for proofreading, Marie Lorimer for compiling the index, and Myriam Megharbi for her help with data permissions.